An Overview of Drooling in Children

Jeyasakthy Saniasiaya
Editor

An Overview of Drooling in Children

Springer

Editor
Jeyasakthy Saniasiaya
Department of Otorhinolaryngology
Universiti Malaya
Kuala Lumpur, Kuala Lumpur, Malaysia

ISBN 978-981-92-1849-3 ISBN 978-981-92-1850-9 (eBook)
https://doi.org/10.1007/978-981-92-1850-9

This Springer imprint is published by the registered company Springer Nature Singapore Pte Ltd.
The registered company address is: 152 Beach Road, #21-01/04 Gateway East, Singapore 189721, Singapore

To every child who inspires resilience,
and to the parents and caregivers who
embody devotion
May knowledge bring hope, and care bring
transformation.

Preface

Drooling in children is a complex and often underestimated clinical condition that requires a nuanced, individualized approach to diagnosis, assessment, and management. While frequently associated with neurodevelopmental and neuromuscular disorders, drooling presents across a wide spectrum of pediatric populations and demands coordinated multidisciplinary care.

An Overview of Drooling in Children has been developed as a comprehensive yet practical manual to support clinicians, students, and researchers navigating this evolving field. This text brings together current scientific understanding with clinically applicable strategies, bridging pathophysiology, structured assessment, and evidence-based management options.

The book addresses drooling across developmental stages, highlighting key differences in presentation and therapeutic considerations between younger children and adolescents. Special attention is given to children with comorbid conditions, where management often requires tailored modifications and collaborative care. Importantly, a dedicated chapter explores drooling in developmentally normal children, an area that has received limited focused discussion in the existing literature.

Chapters are authored by experienced clinicians and recognized experts who provide up-to-date reviews and practical guidance for diagnostic investigations, longitudinal management, and long-term follow-up. The aim of this manual is not only to synthesize current knowledge but also to offer a structured framework that supports informed clinical decision-making.

We hope that this book will serve as a valuable reference and contribute meaningfully to improving care and quality of life for children affected by drooling.

Kuala Lumpur, Malaysia　　　　Jeyasakthy Saniasiaya

Acknowledgments First and foremost, I am deeply grateful to God for His unwavering guidance and strength at every step of this journey.

I humbly express my deepest gratitude to all my mentors for their wisdom, direction, and steadfast encouragement over the years.

To my husband, Dr. Prakashrao Appareo, you are my anchor and my greatest strength. Your unwavering love, belief, and quiet sacrifices sustain me far beyond what words can convey.

To my parents, in-laws, and family, thank you for your enduring support, patience, and faith in me.

To my students and trainees, you challenge me to think more deeply, strive harder, and lead better. Your curiosity and dedication continually inspire my growth as a clinician, educator, and researcher.

To my co-authors, it is both an honor and a privilege to collaborate with such distinguished colleagues. Your expertise and shared commitment to improving children's lives have profoundly shaped this book.

Jeyasakthy Saniasiaya

Contents

Introduction to Drooling in Paediatric Population

1

Jeyasakthy Saniasiaya and Haytham Kubba

1.1 Introduction

Drooling, also referred to as sialorrhoea or salivary incontinence, can be defined as the unintentional loss of saliva [1]. Drooling has been attributed to the lack of coordinated control of saliva by the muscles of the oral cavity, oropharynx, and tongue. Drooling is considered normal up to the age of 18–24 months, which is parallel to the maturation of oro-motor skills and sensory function.

Drooling can be classified as anterior and posterior drooling. Anterior drooling involves saliva spillage beyond the lower lip and chin, whereas in posterior drooling, saliva spillage is noted through the oropharynx and hypopharynx. Typically, the moment saliva enters the hypopharynx, the sensation of saliva generates a swallowing reflex. If the swallow trigger is delayed or absent, saliva pooling in the laryngopharynx results in posterior drooling, producing a gurgling sound at the back of the throat, coughing, gagging, vomiting, and aspiration [2].

The saliva control process is regarded as a form of perception-action coupling [3]. The sensation of the saliva flowing down the lips is considered essential for the development of saliva control. Salivary continence typically develops in parallel with regular feeding as well as oral-motor control. Drooling in children over 4 years is considered pathological and may be related to a myriad of factors, including oromotor difficulties, sensory processing problems in the oral cavity, and insufficient

J. Saniasiaya (✉)
Department of Otorhinolaryngology, Faculty of Medicine, Universiti Malaya, Kuala Lumpur, Malaysia
e-mail: jeyasakthy@um.edu.my

H. Kubba
University of Glasgow, Glasgow, UK

Royal Hospital for Children, Glasgow, UK
e-mail: haytham.kubba@glasgow.ac.uk

J. Saniasiaya (ed.), *An Overview of Drooling in Children*,
https://doi.org/10.1007/978-981-92-1850-9_1

coupling of sensations with the active swallowing process [4]. Incoordination of the oral and oropharyngeal phases of swallowing causes pooling of saliva in the floor of the mouth, leading to spillage in the former or penetration/aspiration in the latter. Typically, once the pharyngeal phase of swallowing is initiated, a series of protective reflex mechanisms is initiated to protect the airway, including hyolaryngeal exclusion and epiglottis deflection, followed by relaxation of the upper esophageal sphincter. However, if the swallow trigger is absent or delayed, saliva pools in the laryngopharynx, leading to gargling, coughing, choking, gagging, vomiting, and aspiration of saliva [2]. It is worth noting that saliva production is typically normal, unlike in hypersalivation, where it increases [5].

1.2 Epidemiology

The prevalence of drooling in children with neurodevelopmental conditions has been reported to be approximately 40%, predominantly anterior drooling (78%) [6]. Although reports on posterior drooling remain scarce, it is estimated to occur in approximately 10–15% of children with neurodevelopmental conditions [2, 7].

1.3 Aetiology

Chronic drooling is classically seen in children with neurological or a combination of oro-motor and sensory processing disabilities [8]. Drooling is associated with multifactorial causes that impair saliva control. Several notable factors reported include reduced perioral and intraoral sensory awareness, inefficiency of the oropharyngeal phase of swallowing, hypotonia, poor head control, poor posture, and reflux. Besides that, children with anatomical or structural conditions that cause mouth breathing, such as a deviated nasal septum, adenoid hypertrophy, allergic rhinitis, malocclusion, or macroglossia, have been reported to drool. Nonetheless, hypersalivation secondary to medication has been reported among children taking anticonvulsants and antipsychotics. Motor or intellectual impairments have also been attributed to drooling [9].

In contrast, acute drooling in children represents a potentially serious clinical sign that warrants urgent evaluation, as it may indicate an impending airway compromise. In the acute setting, drooling can arise from conditions such as epiglottitis, retropharyngeal abscess, caustic ingestion, foreign body aspiration or impaction, and other causes of upper airway obstruction. These conditions share a common pathophysiological mechanism of inability or reluctance to swallow saliva due to pain, inflammation, or mechanical blockage.

1.4 Impact of Drooling in Children

Poor saliva control has been reported to significantly affect the quality of life of both the child and the parents and caretaker. Anterior drooling can lead to perioral infection, dehydration, and comprehension problems [9]. Drooling can cause skin maceration, requiring the change of bibs and clothes multiple times a day, which results in increased personal care for both the child and the carer. Dripping saliva can damage books, electronic devices such as laptops and mobile phones, and other surfaces. As for posterior drooling, it may lead to aspiration, recurrent chest infections, antibiotic use, multiple hospital admissions, and assisted ventilation due to lung damage. Accumulation of stagnant saliva in the oropharynx and hypopharynx often necessitates repeated suctioning, which can inadvertently cause mucosal trauma, bleeding, and increase the risk of secondary infection.

Drooling substantially impacts a child's interpersonal relationships and social interactions, which often leads to embarrassment, reduced self-esteem, and social withdrawal. As a result, it hinders their ability to participate confidently in school activities, form friendships, and integrate effectively into both educational and community settings. Loss of self-esteem and self-confidence among droolers is a significant issue often overlooked.

1.5 Normal Saliva Control and Physiology

Saliva swallowing involves a highly complex and intricate process encompassing volitional and reflexive actions requiring the integrity of 5 nerves and 30 muscles [10]. Saliva flow typically ranges from 0.5 to 1.5 L per day, with variation depending on environmental stimuli and conditions such as temperature and humidity [11]. Salivary flow in infants is influenced by tooth eruption, dietary changes, and age, whereby it increases as the child grows. A growing child will adapt to changes in salivary flow through implicit motor learning, practice, and refinement [12]. The frequency of swallowing in adults has been reported to be once per minute whilst awake, although little data are available on children [13]. Swallowing saliva has been regarded as an automatic act, although it relies on the sensation of feeling saliva accumulation at the floor of the mouth, followed by movement of the tongue to transfer it to the oropharynx.

Saliva is produced by three main paired salivary glands, submandibular, parotid, and sublingual glands, as well as the minor salivary glands. The parotid glands are the largest salivary gland, which delivers saliva through the Stensen's duct, which penetrates the buccal mucosa opposite the upper second molar. The submandibular glands, located in the posterior part of the floor of the mouth, have ducts that drain saliva underneath the tongue, lateral to the lingual frenulum. The smallest among the major salivary glands, the sublingual glands, are located in the floor of the mouth and enter the oral cavity through a series of small ducts opening under the tongue. Collectively, the three paired major salivary glands produce approximately 92 95% of the total saliva volume [14]. The minor salivary glands, which are located mainly in the buccal, labial, and palatal areas and the base of the tongue, produce the remaining saliva.

At rest, the submandibular gland produces approximately 65–70% of total saliva production. Typically, the submandibular gland produces watery saliva. The parotid gland produces nearly 20% of the total saliva content, producing watery content of secretion, whilst the sublingual gland contributes almost 5% of the thicker saliva content. Minor salivary gland collectively contributes another 5–10% of the total salivary content.

Salivary glands are controlled by both the parasympathetic and sympathetic nervous systems. The salivary glands are regulated by the parasympathetic and sympathetic nervous systems, which are influenced by external stimuli such as vision, smell, and taste.

The parasympathetic fibers, which originate in the pons and medulla of the midbrain, synapse in the otic ganglia for the parotid gland and submandibular ganglia for the submandibular and sublingual glands. Acetylcholine is released at the nerve endings of postganglionic parasympathetic fibers, which subsequently directly stimulates the secretion of saliva. Saliva secretion of the minor salivary gland, on the contrary, is less dependent on neuronal control, which spontaneously and continuously secretes a small volume of saliva. Minor salivary glands are continuously produced even during sleep, when the major glands are at rest, and are essential for lubrication and surface protection to ensure continuous oral comfort [14].

1.6 Importance of Saliva

Saliva is essential for maintaining a homeostatic microenvironment within the oral cavity, at rest as well as during swallowing, enabling optimal acid-base and bacterial balance and ensuring bacteriostatic and bactericidal effects. Lubrication of the oral cavity is vital for maintaining dental and oral hygiene and for facilitating swallowing. It is also crucial for the early stages of carbohydrate digestion. Excessive and insufficient saliva may be detrimental, as optimal salivary balance is essential in maintaining oral and upper airway health. Saliva plays a vital role in lubrication, digestion, protection against infection, and preservation of mucosal integrity, making its regulation crucial in children with a drooling problem.

1.7 Assessment

Assessment of a drooling child should begin with a meticulous clinical evaluation that integrates both functional and anatomical considerations. A thorough anamnesis should explore the onset, duration, and frequency of drooling, together with aggravating and relieving factors such as feeding, posture, or fatigue. The presence of associated symptoms, including dysphagia, choking episodes, speech delay, nasal obstruction, and reflux, helps to delineate whether drooling is primarily due to excessive saliva production or impaired saliva control. History should include developmental milestones, neurological history, and prior interventions, as these often provide critical insight into the underlying pathophysiology.

A systematic physical examination begins with observation of the child's posture, facial tone, and alertness. Pay close attention to lip closure, mouth breathing, and head control as these influence saliva pooling and clearance. Assessment of the orofacial region should include inspection of the lips, tongue, palate, dentition, and gingiva to detect malocclusion, macroglossia, or poor oral hygiene. Evaluation of oral-motor skills, including tongue mobility, coordination, and strength, provides valuable information on functional deficits. The state of nasal patency and palatal function should be assessed, as nasal obstruction or velopharyngeal incompetence may compound anterior drooling.

Neurological examination is essential to assess tone, coordination, cranial nerve function, and swallowing reflexes. Observation of spontaneous swallowing frequency and ability to manage secretions helps determine the severity of dysfunction. The presence of perioral skin irritation, fissuring, or odour indicates chronic drooling and its dermatological sequelae. Validated scales such as the Drooling Severity and Frequency Scale (DSFS), Teacher's Drooling Scale (TDS), or visual analogue ratings may be applied. Where feasible, instrumental assessments, including videofluoroscopic swallow study (VFSS) and fiberoptic endoscopic evaluation of swallowing (FEES), can be used to determine the site and mechanism of dysfunction.

A comprehensive assessment that integrates these findings with multidisciplinary input is crucial to delineate the relative contributions of structural, sensory, and motor factors, thereby guiding the formulation of an individualized management plan for each child.

1.8 Management

The main aim of intervention when managing a child with drooling is to reduce saliva spillage or aspiration, thereby improving the child's overall quality of life and reducing complications. A myriad of non-pharmacological, pharmacological, and surgical interventions are widely available. Non-pharmacological interventions include behavioural therapies and oro-motor therapy, whilst pharmacological treatment aims to reduce saliva rate and frequency and mainly includes anticholinergics. As for surgical intervention, salivary duct clipping, salivary gland excision, and rerouting/interposition of the salivary duct have been widely practised with promising results.

1.9 Multidisciplinary Care

A multidisciplinary team is fundamental when managing a child with drooling, given its multifactorial nature, which rarely resolves through a single intervention. Effective management typically involves an interdisciplinary team comprising paediatric otorhinolaryngologists, speech and language therapists, paediatric dentists, rehabilitation specialists, and child psychologists or counsellors. The involvement of a multidisciplinary team enables a holistic approach, integrating medical, functional, and psychosocial perspectives to craft an individualized management plan that optimizes each child's function, participation, and quality of life.

References

1. Johnson H, King J, Reddihough DS. Children with sialorrhoea in the absence of neurological abnormalities. Child Care Health Dev. 2001;27(6):591–602.
2. Jongerius PH, van Hulst K, van den Hoogen FJ, Rotteveel JJ. The treatment of posterior drooling by botulinum toxin in a child with cerebral palsy. J Pediatr Gastroenterol Nutr. 2005;41:351–3.
3. Rotem-Kohavi N, Hilderman CG, Liu A, Makan N, Wang JZ, Virji-Babul N. Network analysis of perception-action coupling in infants. Front Hum Neurosci. 2014;8:209.
4. Burgmayer S, Jung H. Hypersalivation in severe mental retardation. Int J Rehabil Res. 1983;6(2):193–6.
5. Little SA, Kubba H, Hussain SS. An evidence-based approach to the child who drools saliva. Clin Otolaryngol. 2009;34(3):236–9. https://doi.org/10.1111/j.1749-4486.2009.01917.x. PMID: 19531173.
6. Tahmassebi JF, Curzon ME. Prevalence of drooling in children with cerebral palsy attending special schools. Dev Med Child Neurol. 2003;45:613–7.
7. van Hulst CC. Oral motor performance in children with neurodevelopmental disabilities-about dysphagia and drooling. Doctoral dissertation. 2019.
8. Blasco PA. Management of drooling: 10 years after the Consortium on Drooling, 1990. Dev Med Child Neurol. 2002;44:778–81.
9. Daniel SJ, Fayoux P, Bateman N, Boudewyns A, Brigger M, Chan CY, Chan K, Cheng A, Conley S, Kubba H, Lambert EM, Muntz H, Nuss R, Russell J, Rutter M, Schwarz Y, Spratley J, Thevasagayam R, Thompson D, Valika T, Wyatt M. Comprehensive management of anterior drooling: an International Pediatric Otolaryngology Group (IPOG) consensus statement. Int J Pediatr Otorhinolaryngol. 2023;168:111500.
10. Matsuo K, Palmer JB. Anatomy and physiology of feeding and swallowing: normal and abnormal. Phys Med Rehabil Clin N Am. 2008;19(4):691–707, vii. https://doi.org/10.1016/j.pmr.2008.06.001.
11. Humphrey SP, Williamson RT. A review of saliva: normal composition, flow, and function. J Prosthet Dent. 2001;85(2):162–9. https://doi.org/10.1067/mpr.2001.113778. PMID: 11208206.
12. Sheppard JJ. Using motor learning approaches for treating swallowing and feeding disorders: a review. Lang Speech Hear Serv Sch. 2008;39(2):227–36. https://doi.org/10.1044/0161-1461(2008/022). PMID: 18420525.
13. Fairhurst CB, Cockerill H. Management of drooling in children. Arch Dis Childhood Educ Pract. 2011;96(1):25–30.
14. Varga G. Physiology of the salivary glands. Surgery (Oxford). 2012;30(11):578–83.

2 Etiology and Pathophysiology of Drooling in Children

Elisabeth R. Wenneker, Deepak K. Mehta, and Elton M. Lambert

2.1 Introduction

Drooling is the loss of saliva from the oral cavity and is also referred to as ptyalism and sialorrhea [1, 2]. Drooling can be classified as anterior or posterior. Anterior drooling occurs when saliva spills out of the oral cavity onto the lips and face. In contrast, posterior drooling occurs when saliva spills through the oropharynx into the hypopharynx, posing an aspiration risk. Drooling can occur with or without aspiration. The cause of drooling is often multifactorial, related to impaired motor control of the upper aerodigestive tract and uncoordinated oral phase of swallow, rather than hypersalivation [1, 3–7].

Drooling is considered physiologic in infancy and early childhood. In a neurotypical child, drooling improves as oral sensorimotor skills develop around age 18–24 months [1]. However, it is considered abnormal when it occurs after 4 years of age while awake [8, 9]. Pathologic drooling is common in specific pediatric populations, including those with neuromuscular disease such as cerebral palsy. The prevalence of drooling in patients with cerebral palsy is around 44%; however, this number varies widely across studies [10]. Like physiologic drooling, pathologic drooling tends to decrease with age in patients with cerebral palsy [11].

E. R. Wenneker · D. K. Mehta · E. M. Lambert (✉)
Bobby R. Alford Department of Otolaryngology – Head and Neck Surgery, Baylor College of Medicine, Houston, TX, USA

Texas Children's Hospital, Department of Otolaryngology, Houston, TX, USA
e-mail: dkmehta@texaschildrens.org; deepak.mehta@bcm.edu; emashela@texaschildrens.org

J. Saniasiaya (ed.), *An Overview of Drooling in Children*,
https://doi.org/10.1007/978-981-92-1850-9_2

There can be significant side effects of drooling, ranging from mild or inconvenient to severe, with a negative impact on health, psychosocial function, and quality of life for patients and caregivers. Anterior drooling can lead to soiled clothing, resulting in skin breakdown and infection, oral infections, and dehydration. Posterior drooling can lead to aspiration, resulting in recurrent pneumonias, chronic cough, the need for inhaled bronchodilators and corticosteroids, and frequent hospitalizations. Drooling can be associated with speech impairment and has a negative impact on patients' ability to engage with rehabilitation therapies. Drooling is an additional barrier to education due to the inability to share school materials like books and computers [1, 2, 9, 12, 13].

2.2 Normal Salivary Function

Saliva is critical for oral health and the function of oral tissues [14]. It aids in the mechanical cleansing of the mouth, promotes oral homeostasis, supports dental hygiene, and reduces oral odor. It also has bacteriostatic and bactericidal properties. Saliva contributes to the formation of the enamel pellicle, a thin acellular film on tooth surfaces that helps maintain dental health. It also serves as a buffering system to maintain a neutral pH to decrease tooth demineralization [15]. Saliva also plays a role in digestion by lubricating the food bolus formed in the oral cavity, and it contains amylase, which initiates the digestion of starches [9].

Six major salivary glands produce about 90% of saliva, while the remainder is produced by hundreds of minor salivary glands throughout the oral cavity and pharynx [9]. Unstimulated daily saliva is primarily produced by the submandibular glands (71%), followed by the parotid glands (25%) and sublingual glands (3–4%) [16]. However, stimulated saliva production mainly comes from the paired parotid glands; stimulated saliva contributes up to 90% of the average daily production. Salivary flow rate is variable, but tends to stabilize around age 15 [17]. Salivary flow ranges from 0.3 mL/min unstimulated to 7 mL/min stimulated in adults, with an average daily production of 1000–1500 mL [16]. There is a lack of data on salivary flow in children.

Salivation is primarily controlled by the parasympathetic nervous system with some contribution from the sympathetic nervous system. The superior and inferior salivatory nuclei are in the pons and medulla, respectively; they are triggered by chewing as well as gustatory and olfactory stimuli. Preganglionic parasympathetic fibers from the superior salivatory nucleus travel along the chorda tympani branch of cranial nerve VII, prior to joining the lingual branch of cranial nerve VII and synapsing at the submandibular ganglion. The postganglionic fibers then stimulate submandibular and sublingual secretion. Preganglionic parasympathetic fibers from the inferior salivatory nucleus travel along cranial nerve IX and synapse at the otic ganglion. The postganglionic fibers travel along the auriculotemporal nerve to stimulate parotid secretion. Sympathetic innervation causes contraction of muscle fibers around salivary ducts to regulate the flow of saliva [9].

2.3 Etiology and Pathophysiology

Drooling is distinguished by frequency and direction. It can be constant, frequent, or occasional and classified as either anterior or posterior. Anterior drooling causes more social stigma and psychosocial problems than medical problems, whereas posterior drooling often leads to aspiration and progression of chronic lung disease [1, 2]. Patients can present with both anterior and posterior drooling. Risk factors for drooling include generalized neuromuscular dysfunction, impaired oral motor and sensory function, structural abnormalities of the aerodigestive tract, and iatrogenic causes like medication side effects.

Generalized neuromuscular dysfunction from cerebral palsy and muscular dystrophy is a common risk factor for drooling [9]. Hypotonia can lead to poor head control and poor posture, which further contribute to drooling [1, 2, 18]. Many studies have shown that pathologic drooling in patients with cerebral palsy is caused by oral motor and sensory dysfunction. This manifests as decreased frequency of swallow, difficulty initiating swallow, saliva pooling in the dependent portions of the mouth, and inability to transport saliva to the pharynx [4, 12, 19, 20]. These patients also have uncoordinated tongue movements and high tone and spasticity of the pharynx [7]. There may be a relationship between oral sensation and drooling in patients with cerebral palsy as well [21]. The sensory dysfunction decreases a patient's ability to recognize saliva pooling in the oral cavity, and motor dysfunction impacts a patient's ability to manage their saliva.

Upper airway obstruction and/or structural abnormalities of the aerodigestive tract can lead to mouth breathing, which leads to increased drooling [1]. Normal swallowing can occur only when the jaw is stable and the mouth is closed, so malocclusion and open mouth posture cause drooling [4, 22, 23]. Tooth eruption, gingivitis, and teething are other contributing factors [1, 18], as well as adenotonsillar hypertrophy, nasal obstruction, macroglossia, and ankyloglossia. It is thought that reflux and allergies may also play a role in drooling [2].

Finally, there are medications that cause increased drooling due to increased production of saliva. This includes certain antiepileptics and antipsychotics, including clobazam, clozapine, and topiramate. It has been shown that tapering off these medications can improve drooling [1, 2, 24, 25].

2.4 Assessment

Evaluating a patient with pathologic drooling requires obtaining a detailed history and focused physical exam, as well as several functional assessment tools. It is essential to determine the onset, duration, and frequency of a child's drooling. For some, it may be constant, frequent, or occasional [1]. The provider should inquire about any comorbid symptoms, such as coughing, choking, a wet voice, dysphagia, allergies, or reflux and document the frequency and severity of any respiratory illnesses. A review of the patient's medications should also be done to identify any iatrogenic causes of drooling.

Physical exam should include a neurological, craniofacial, and oral cavity exam. Assessing their dental hygiene and the presence of occlusion or malocclusion is critical as well. Providers should ensure to document the patient's overall posture and whether the patient is hypotonic. Flexible nasopharyngoscopy can provide vital information to determine whether there is any upper airway obstruction, like adenoid hypertrophy, that may contribute to open mouth posturing and drooling.

Additionally, more invasive testing may provide important diagnostic information when assessing drooling. Dysphagia frequently occurs in patients with drooling, and so various instruments can be used to assess swallowing. These include fiberoptic endoscopic evaluation of swallowing (FEES), video fluoroscopic swallow study (VFSS), and modified Evans' blue dye test for patients who are nil per os (NPO). Suppose there are concerns for anatomic differences in the larynx that may contribute to posterior drooling and aspiration, such as a laryngeal cleft or tracheoesophageal fistula. In that case, it may be prudent to perform a direct laryngoscopy in the operating room. Additional tests for tracing saliva include radionuclide salivagram with technetium 99m sulfur colloid [26].

Evaluating and treating patients who drool requires multidisciplinary care from the pediatrician, otolaryngologist, speech language pathologist, neurologist, and pulmonologist who are treating the child. Engaging the patient's caregivers to determine the best management and treatment options is imperative to ensure the best outcomes for the patient.

2.5 Conclusion

The etiology of drooling is multifactorial and requires a multidisciplinary approach for optimal evaluation and management. Pathologic drooling is common in patients with cerebral palsy. Oral motor and sensory dysfunction in conjunction with upper airway obstruction and malocclusion result in drooling, which is often comorbid with feeding and swallowing difficulties. The medical and psychosocial side effects of drooling can have a profound negative impact on both the patient and the caregiver. It is important to understand the modifiable risk factors for this condition in order to best treat it.

References

1. Daniel SJ, Fayoux P, Bateman N, et al. Comprehensive management of anterior drooling: an International Pediatric Otolaryngology Group (IPOG) consensus statement. Int J Pediatr Otorhinolaryngol. 2023;168:111500. https://doi.org/10.1016/j.ijporl.2023.111500.
2. Hughes A, Lambert EM. Drooling and aspiration of saliva. Otolaryngol Clin N Am. 2022;55(6):1181–94. https://doi.org/10.1016/j.otc.2022.07.007.
3. Sarvas E, Webb J, Landrigan-Ossar M, et al. Oral health care for children and youth with developmental disabilities: clinical report. Pediatrics. 2024;154(2):e2024067603. https://doi.org/10.1542/peds.2024-067603.

4. Iammatteo PA, Trombly C, Luecke L. The effect of mouth closure on drooling and speech. Am J Occup Ther. 1990;44(8):686–91. https://doi.org/10.5014/ajot.44.8.686.
5. Tahmassebi JF, Curzon MEJ. The cause of drooling in children with cerebral palsy – hypersalivation or swallowing defect? Int J Paediatr Dent. 2003;13(2):106–11. https://doi.org/10.1046/j.1365-263x.2003.00439.x.
6. Lespargot A, Langevin MF, Muller S, Guillemont S. Swallowing disturbances associated with drooling in cerebral-palsied children. Dev Med Child Neurol. 1993;35(4):298–304. https://doi.org/10.1111/j.1469-8749.1993.tb11641.x.
7. Ekedahl C, Månsson I, Sandberg N. Swallowing dysfunction in the brain-damaged with drooling. Acta Otolaryngol (Stockh). 1974;78(1–2):141–9. https://doi.org/10.3109/00016487409126339.
8. Brei TJ. Management of drooling. Semin Pediatr Neurol. 2003;10(4):265–70. https://doi.org/10.1016/s1071-9091(03)00072-x.
9. Hockstein NG, Samadi DS, Gendron K, Handler SD. Sialorrhea: a management challenge. Am Fam Physician. 2004;69(11):2628–34.
10. Speyer R, Cordier R, Kim JH, Cocks N, Michou E, Wilkes-Gillan S. Prevalence of drooling, swallowing, and feeding problems in cerebral palsy across the lifespan: a systematic review and meta-analyses. Dev Med Child Neurol. 2019;61(11):1249–58. https://doi.org/10.1111/dmcn.14316.
11. Hegde AM, Pani SC. Drooling of saliva in children with cerebral palsy-etiology, prevalence, and relationship to salivary flow rate in an Indian population. Spec Care Dent. 2009;29(4):163–8. https://doi.org/10.1111/j.1754-4505.2009.00085.x.
12. Goode RL, Smith RA. The surgical management of sialorrhea. Laryngoscope. 1970;80(7):1078–89. https://doi.org/10.1288/00005537-197007000-00006.
13. Wilkie TF. The problem of drooling in cerebral palsy: a surgical approach. Can J Surg J Can Chir. 1967;10(1):60–7.
14. Schubert MM, Izutsu KT. Iatrogenic causes of salivary gland dysfunction. J Dent Res. 1987;66 Spec No:680–8. https://doi.org/10.1177/00220345870660S213.
15. Lynge Pedersen AM, Belstrøm D. The role of natural salivary defences in maintaining a healthy oral microbiota. J Dent. 2019;80(Suppl 1):S3–S12. https://doi.org/10.1016/j.jdent.2018.08.010.
16. Flint PW, Haughey B, Lund V, et al. Cummings otolaryngology: head and neck surgery. 7th ed. Elsevier; 2020. https://www.clinicalkey.com/#!/content/book/3-s2.0-B9780323611794000818. Accessed 29 July 2025.
17. Humphrey SP, Williamson RT. A review of saliva: normal composition, flow, and function. J Prosthet Dent. 2001;85(2):162–9. https://doi.org/10.1067/mpr.2001.113778.
18. Reid SM, McCutcheon J, Reddihough DS, Johnson H. Prevalence and predictors of drooling in 7- to 14-year-old children with cerebral palsy: a population study. Dev Med Child Neurol. 2012;54(11):1032–6. https://doi.org/10.1111/j.1469-8749.2012.04382.x.
19. Lawrence R, Bateman N. Surgical management of the drooling child. Curr Otorhinolaryngol Rep. 2018;6(1):99–106. https://doi.org/10.1007/s40136-018-0188-2.
20. Sochaniwskyj AE, Koheil RM, Bablich K, Milner M, Kenny DJ. Oral motor functioning, frequency of swallowing and drooling in normal children and in children with cerebral palsy. Arch Phys Med Rehabil. 1986;67(12):866–74.
21. Weiss-Lambrou R, Tétreault S, Dudley J. The relationship between oral sensation and drooling in persons with cerebral palsy. Am J Occup Ther. 1989;43(3):155–61. https://doi.org/10.5014/ajot.43.3.155.
22. Ray SA, Bundy AC, Nelson DL. Decreasing drooling through techniques to facilitate mouth closure. Am J Occup Ther. 1983;37(11):749–53. https://doi.org/10.5014/ajot.37.11.749.
23. Franklin DL, Luther F, Curzon ME. The prevalence of malocclusion in children with cerebral palsy. Eur J Orthod. 1996;18(6):637–43. https://doi.org/10.1093/ejo/18.6.637.
24. Yam WKL, Yang HLC, Abdullah V, Chan CYL. Management of drooling for children with neurological problems in Hong Kong. Brain Dev. 2006;28(1):24–9. https://doi.org/10.1016/j.braindev.2005.03.008.

25. Donegan S, Dixon P, Hemming K, Tudur-Smith C, Marson A. A systematic review of placebo-controlled trials of topiramate: how useful is a multiple-indications review for evaluating the adverse events of an antiepileptic drug? Epilepsia. 2015;56(12):1910–20. https://doi.org/10.1111/epi.13209.
26. Simons JP, Rubinstein EN, Mandell DL. Clinical predictors of aspiration on radionuclide salivagrams in children. Arch Otolaryngol Head Neck Surg. 2008;134(9):941–4. https://doi.org/10.1001/archotol.134.9.941.

Clinical Evaluation and Investigations of Drooling in Children

3

Kalliopi Argyriou and Ravi Thevasagayam

3.1 Introduction

Drooling refers to the involuntary spillage or overflow of saliva from the oral cavity beyond the lips, or its pooling and overflow into the oropharynx with potential risk of aspiration [1, 2]. In infancy and early toddlerhood, drooling is commonly seen as part of normal development; with maturation of oromotor control and swallowing reflexes, most children are able to achieve salivary "continence". Salivary control is normally established by 15–18 months of age but it is not uncommon for the drooling to persist, especially in boys, until about 6 or 7 years old. This may simply be due to lack to social awareness, and if developmentally normal, parents can be reassured that the children will "outgrow" this. Parents may have looked online and seen that treatments are available, but they should be advised that treatments can cause significant morbidity and are generally reserved for cases with neurological comorbidities [3].

Chronic or persistent drooling is particularly common in children with neurodevelopmental disabilities such as cerebral palsy (CP), neuromuscular disease, genetic syndromes, or developmental delay [4, 5]. The reported prevalence of drooling in CP varies widely, between 10% and up to 58% depending on cohort and severity [4].

The clinical and psychosocial burden is substantial. Drooling may cause skin maceration, perioral dermatitis, dental caries, malodour, frequent clothing changes, social stigma, reduced self-esteem, increased caregiver burden, and, in cases of posterior drooling, risk of silent aspiration, recurrent chest infections, chronic lung disease, and even life-threatening respiratory morbidity [4, 6].

Drooling may be considered to be *anterior* when there is visible saliva loss beyond the lip margins and *posterior* when saliva spills through the oropharynx into

K. Argyriou · R. Thevasagayam (✉)
Sheffield Children's Hospital, Sheffield, UK
e-mail: kalliopi.argyriou@nhs.net; ravi.theva@nhs.net

J. Saniasiaya (ed.), *An Overview of Drooling in Children*,
https://doi.org/10.1007/978-981-92-1850-9_3

the hypopharynx. The main implications of anterior drooling are related to social impact, perioral soreness, and increased burden of care (wiping, replacement of bibs and clothes). Posterior drooling poses an increased risk of aspiration and may have a significant impact of the child's respiratory health. It may also be indicative of a potentially unsafe swallowing function.

Given the heterogeneity of underlying causes and the broad spectrum of clinical impact, from minor anterior dribble to life-threatening aspiration, a structured, multidisciplinary evaluation is essential. Such an approach aims to:

- Define the drooling type (anterior/posterior/mixed), the severity, and the impact
- Identify modifiable contributors (anatomical, postural, neuromotor, sensory)
- Detect aspiration risk
- Guide tailored management (behavioural, medical, surgical)

3.2 Why Children Drool: Pathophysiology and Aetiology

Although the term "sialorrhoea" may imply hypersalivation, the saliva production in children is within physiological range, and overt hypersalivation is comparatively rare [1]. In paediatric and neurodisability populations, drooling is almost always due to impaired oromotor control, reduced swallowing frequency, poor posture, sensory deficits, and craniofacial/dental/airway pathology, rather than increased saliva production per se [1, 7].

Key pathophysiological factors include:

- Poor lip seal, weak tongue and lip control, inability to maintain closed mouth posture
- Reduced frequency of spontaneous swallowing, decreased oropharyngeal sensation, and impaired motor coordination of the tongue, jaw, and palate
- Postural instability: poor head or trunk control
- Craniofacial anomalies and dental malocclusion that interfere with effective lip closure or oral containment
- Airway problems (nasal obstruction, enlarged adenoids/tonsils, macroglossia)
- Neurological or neuromuscular disorders affecting swallowing (dysphagia), bulbar function, or sensorimotor integration [1, 4, 7]

Because of this multifactorial origin, drooling may occur in isolation or together with swallowing dysfunction (dysphagia) and may manifest as anterior drooling, posterior drooling, or more commonly a combination of both [1, 4].

3.3 Clinical Assessment

A comprehensive clinical assessment remains the cornerstone of drooling evaluation. In many children, especially those with anterior drooling only, a detailed history and clinical examination may be sufficient to define the drooling phenotype and guide conservative management, without the need for immediate instrumental studies [1, 7].

History should include:

- Age of onset and trajectory: when did drooling start, has it worsened or changed over time
- Contexts and triggers: awake vs sleep, feeding vs rest, concentration (writing, school), excitement, fatigue, posture positioning, activity
- Feeding and swallowing: texture of diet, difficulties in chewing or swallowing, prolonged mealtimes, coughing or choking during or after feeds, need for suctioning, refusal of food, fatigue with meals
- Respiratory history: recurrent lower respiratory tract infections, pneumonia, hospitalisations, desaturations, need for suctioning, ventilator or tracheostomy dependence, airway issues, noisy breathing, wet voice, gurgly breathing
- Neurological and developmental background: underlying diagnoses, neurological symptoms (tone, motor impairment, movement disorders), developmental delay, communication ability, medications (especially those that might increase salivation)
- Psychosocial impact: social embarrassment, self-esteem, participation in school or social activities, caregiver burden, hygiene problems, skin breakdown, distress [2, 3, 7]

Physical examination should include:

- Assessment of posture: head control, trunk/seating (for wheelchair users), neck alignment, habitual head position (chin up/down), alignment in sitting/standing
- Oral anatomy: lip seal (closed mouth at rest), dental malocclusion, oral hygiene, jaw control, palate and tongue posture and mobility, presence of macroglossia
- Airway patency: nasal obstruction, enlarged tonsils and adenoids, history of mouth-breathing, sleep-disordered breathing
- Observation of saliva: pooling in mouth, frequency of drooling, ability to clear drool, chin wiping, bib/clothing changes
- Neurological examination: tone, reflexes, bulbar function, cranial nerve function, involuntary movements, swallowing reflexes, ability to protect airway when swallowing and with secretions

Severity and impact assessment should use structured tools where possible: drooling frequency/severity scales, bib-counting or clothing-change diaries, caregiver questionnaires assessing quality of life, social participation, hygiene burden, and caregiver time. Several scales have been used in the literature which provide useful baseline and outcome measures [3–5]. A recent COSMIN-based review recommended a combination of tools [8]. Some of the commonly used scales are listed below.

- *Thomas-Stonell & Greenberg Drooling Severity and Frequency Scale (DSFS)*—5-point severity × 4-point frequency [9]
- *Drooling Quotient (DQ)*—observational count of drooling episodes over fixed time (e.g. 5 or 10 min), often used in research [8, 10]
- *Drooling Rating Scale/Drooling Impact Scale (DIS)*—focus on functional impact and change after interventions [10]
- *Teacher's Drooling Scale/modified TDS*—rating scale used by carers/teachers [8]

3.4 When to Escalate: Indications for Instrumental Investigations

In children with only anterior drooling, no signs of aspiration or respiratory involvement, and limited functional impact, conservative management may begin without further investigations although regular reassessment is advised. Instrumental swallowing and aspiration assessment should be considered when one or more of the following are present [4, 11]:

- Clinical features suggestive of posterior drooling or salivary aspiration: wet/gurgly voice, noisy breathing, frequent choking or coughing (especially during or after feeding), need for frequent suctioning of secretions, recurrent or chronic respiratory infections, desaturation or apnoea episodes, tracheostomy or ventilator dependence, unexplained lung radiological changes.
- Feeding difficulties: prolonged mealtimes, coughing/choking on thin liquids or saliva, fatigue, poor weight gain, malnutrition, refusal of certain textures, anticipated need for texture modification.
- Planning of irreversible interventions (e.g. surgical salivary gland duct ligation, salivary duct diversion, radiation): baseline swallow and airway assessment is essential to guide decision-making and to monitor risk.
- Complex or mixed aetiology: combination of neuromotor impairment, craniofacial/dental/airway structural abnormalities, neuromuscular disease.
- Unclear diagnosis.
- Previous conservative therapy failure.

Thus, a stepwise, judicious, and multidisciplinary decision-making process should determine who needs further investigations [12, 13].

3.5 Instrumental Diagnostics

Each of the available investigations has specific indications and limitations; therefore, a combination of tests is often required. The diagnostic workup should be guided by the clinical question (swallow physiology, secretion management, aspiration risk), the child's cooperation and condition, and the available resources.

3.5.1 Videofluoroscopic Swallow Study (VFSS)/Modified Barium Swallow

VFSS remains the most widely used dynamic swallowing study in paediatrics [12–14]. It involves ingestion of radiopaque contrast (barium) in various textures and viscosities under real-time fluoroscopy. The VFSS allows visualization of all the phases of swallowing, the bolus transit, the airway protection, and the effect of compensatory strategies [12, 14, 16]. Aspiration may be demonstrated with clear ingress of contrast onto the vocal cords (penetration) or overt aspiration (Fig. 3.1).

Strengths:

- Provides comprehensive view of swallow biomechanics including oral, pharyngeal, oesophageal phases [12, 16]
- Helps to guide feeding recommendations: safe textures, posture, pacing, compensatory strategies
- Useful in planning oral vs enteral feeding and in pre-surgical evaluation

Limitations:

- Requires child cooperation; difficult for many children with severe neurodisability or cognitive impairment
- Exposure to ionizing radiation; may limit repeated studies
- Provides only a brief "snapshot"; may miss intermittent or low-volume aspiration, especially of saliva rather than food/liquid boluses
- Does not assess secretion management per se (i.e. pooling or constant saliva flow), or airway clearance of secretions

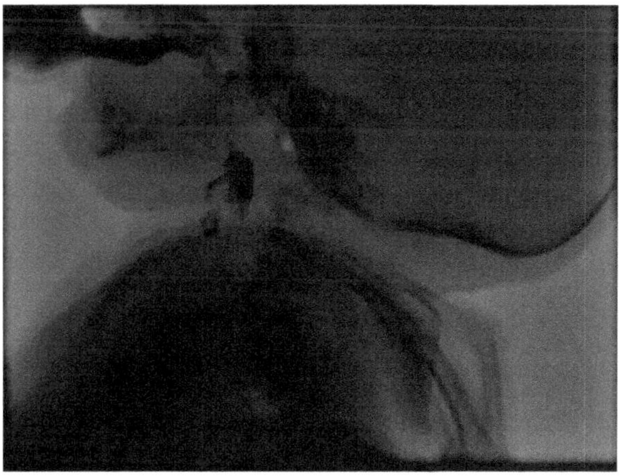

Fig. 3.1 Evidence of aspiration on VFSS

Because of these limitations, a negative VFSS does not rule out ongoing salivary aspiration, particularly in children with complex neurodisability, secretion pooling, or tracheostomy dependence [4, 7, 16].

3.5.2 Flexible Endoscopic Evaluation of Swallowing (FEES)

FEES is increasingly used in children for evaluation of swallowing safety, especially of secretion management and saliva aspiration [13, 15]. A flexible paediatric nasendoscope is passed transnasally into the hypopharynx and allows direct observation of the swallowing process, along with any secretion pooling before, during, and after swallowing (food, fluid, saliva) in real time. Clear aspiration and penetration of coloured food material may be visualised (Fig. 3.2).

Strengths:

- No ionizing radiation; safer for repeated assessments and useful in chronic conditions [12, 13].
- Direct visualization of airway anatomy, secretion pooling, penetration/aspiration of secretions or thin fluids; critical when concern centres on saliva or secretion management [15].
- Can be performed in real-life setting (bedside, usual feeding posture, wheelchair, tracheostomy in situ) [13].

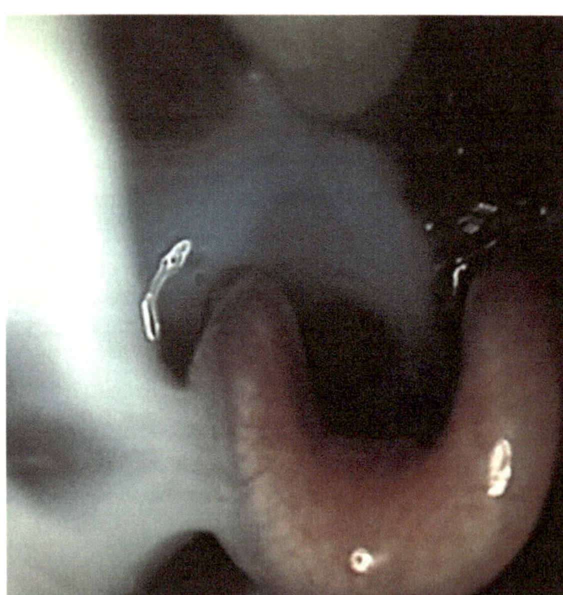

Fig. 3.2 Aspiration viewed during FEES

Limitations:

- Does not visualize the oral and oesophageal phases.
- "White-out" during the swallow (when pharyngeal walls close around endoscope) may obscure the exact moment of aspiration, making detection of penetration/aspiration more challenging.
- Requires skilled personnel (SLT + ENT/trained endoscopist).
- May be poorly tolerated (gag, laryngospasm).
- Aspiration events outside the study period (intermittent aspiration) may be missed; a negative FEES does not exclude risk.

Despite these limitations, FEES is often the more pragmatic choice for children with significant neurodisability, secretion issues, tracheostomy, and poor cooperation and for chronic conditions requiring long-term monitoring [13, 15].

3.5.3 Radionuclide Salivagram/Scintigraphy

Salivagram involves administration of a small radiotracer with saliva-like consistency into the oral cavity followed by serial imaging over time (often 20–60 min) to detect whether labelled saliva enters the airway. This modality is mainly used in children with suspected chronic or intermittent saliva aspiration (posterior drooling), including those with CP, neuromuscular disease, tracheostomy, or ventilator dependence, although it is now not used very often [16].

3.5.4 Additional Investigations

Because drooling may be secondary to or exacerbated by anatomical or neurological factors, additional assessments are often indicated, particularly when there are red flags or the aetiology is unclear:

- *ENT/Airway Review*: Nasendoscopy or flexible nasopharyngoscopy to assess airway patency, nasal obstruction, adenoid/tonsillar hypertrophy, macroglossia, laryngeal structural abnormalities, vocal cord function, pooling secretions, airway protection mechanisms. This is important in children with mouth-breathing, obstructive sleep symptoms, tracheostomy, or chronic secretion management issues [7, 15].
- *Dental/Orthodontic/Craniofacial Assessment*: To identify dental malocclusion, open bite, macroglossia, poor lip seal and jaw abnormalities that impair oral containment. Correcting structural contributors can reduce drooling and improve oral control; in some cases, it may reduce dependence on more invasive therapies [1, 4].
- *Neurological/Neuromuscular/Neuroimaging Assessment*: For children with unexplained drooling, complex neurodisability, developmental delay, neuromuscular signs, progressive symptoms further investigation with brain MRI scan, neurometabolic/genetic testing and neuromuscular studies (e.g. EMG) may elu-

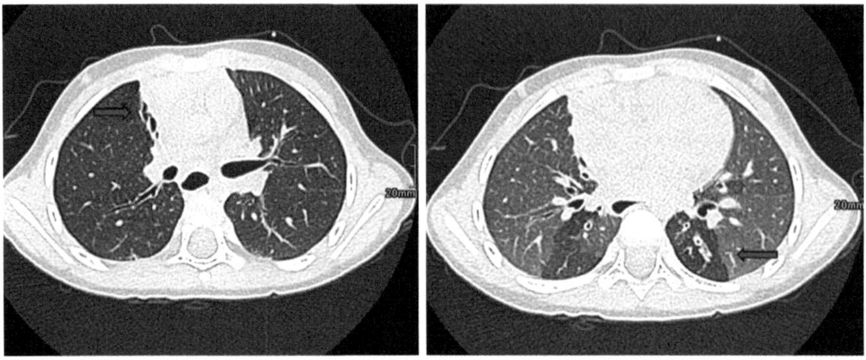

Fig. 3.3 CT scan images with evidence of chronic aspiration: bronchial wall thickening and partial collapse of the anterior segment of the right upper lobe. Focal areas of air trapping involving the lower lobes

cidate underlying diagnosis and guide long-term management. While these investigations do not directly assess swallow physiology, they are often essential for comprehensive care planning [1, 4].

- *Imaging*: Chest x-ray and CT scanning may show chronic lung changes in keeping with aspiration (atelectasis, bronchiectasis) (Fig. 3.3).
- *Bronchoalveolar lavage (BAL)*: Performed via flexible bronchoscopy, the BAL can provide a useful information about the lower airway. In children with chronic respiratory symptoms (recurrent pneumonia, cough, "wet" secretions, or unexplained lung changes), BAL fluid can be analysed for biomarkers such as salivary amylase, pepsin, low-molecular-weight hyaluronan (LMW-HA), as well as Lipid-laden macrophages, which may indicate aspiration of oropharyngeal or gastric contents [17, 18]. Detection of these biomarkers in BAL increases the likelihood that at least intermittent aspiration is occurring, even when "classic" swallowing studies are unremarkable.

3.6 Integrated, Stepwise Decision-Making: A Suggested Clinical Algorithm

Based on best current practice [7, 11, 15]. and the strengths and limitations of available diagnostic modalities, the following stepwise, multidisciplinary, individualised approach is recommended:

1. *Initial Clinical Evaluation*
    - Comprehensive history (feeding, drooling, respiratory, neurological, social impact)
    - Physical, oromotor, airway, dental, and posture/positioning examination
    - Baseline functional and impact assessment (severity/frequency scales, caregiver questionnaire, bib-counting, etc.)

2. *Classification (After Initial Assessment)*
    - Anterior drooling (visible saliva spillage)
    - Suspicion of posterior drooling/salivary aspiration (based on history: gurgly voice, wet breathing, recurrent chest infections, need for suctioning, tracheostomy, or other red flags)
    - Mixed: anterior and posterior drooling
3. *Need for Instrumental/Additional Investigations.*
    - If only anterior drooling, minimal impact, no aspiration or respiratory features → begin conservative management (oromotor therapy, posture, hygiene, dental/ENT review), monitor + reassess periodically
    - If suspicion of aspiration/posterior drooling, feeding difficulties, respiratory disease, planned invasive therapy, complex aetiology → proceed to instrumental and other investigations (VFSS/FEES/salivagram + ENT/dental/neurological as indicated)
4. *Select Appropriate Investigations Based on Clinical Context*
    - *VFSS*: if swallow mechanics/bolus transit need evaluation, and child can cooperate
    - *FEES*: if secretion management/saliva pooling/aspiration risk is the primary concern, if child cannot tolerate VFSS, or if repeated assessments are anticipated
    - *Salivagram*: if there is suspicion of chronic/intermittent salivary aspiration, particularly in severely disabled children, tracheostomy, ventilator-dependence, recurrent pneumonia, or when VFSS and FEES are inconclusive or not feasible
    - *ENT/airway/airway imaging/nasendoscopy, dental/craniofacial assessment, neuroimaging or neuromuscular workup*, as clinically indicated
5. *Integration—Multidimensional Phenotyping*

    After investigations, synthesise data into a "child profile" including: drooling type (anterior/posterior/mixed), severity and frequency, impact (functional/social/caregiver burden), swallow safety (bolus and secretion), airway status, structural/anatomical factors, neurological diagnosis, respiratory status, and feeding ability.
6. *Shared Decision-Making and Management Planning*

    Use the drooling type to guide discussions with caregivers (and child, where appropriate) about goals (comfort, hygiene, social participation, nutrition/hydration, respiratory safety), and to tailor interventions, from least invasive (behavioural therapy, oral-motor exercises, posture, dental/ENT correction) to more invasive (anticholinergic therapy, botulinum toxin, surgical duct ligation/diversion), with periodic reassessment.
7. *Follow-Up and Re-evaluation*

    Because drooling and swallowing status may change over time (growth, neurological regression, motor deterioration, structural changes), periodic reassessment (clinical, functional, instrumental as indicated) is essential. In children with high aspiration risk, regular respiratory follow up and swallow assessment is particularly important.

This structured, stepwise algorithm ensures that children are neither over-investigated nor undertreated and that interventions are tailored, safe, and evidence-based.

3.7 Conclusion

Drooling (sialorrhoea) in children is a common, multifactorial condition, especially encountered in the context of neurodevelopmental or neuromuscular disorders. Its clinical presentation ranges widely, from minor anterior drooling with limited impact to posterior drooling with silent aspiration, chronic respiratory disease and significant morbidity. A structured, stepwise, multidisciplinary evaluation, beginning with careful history and detailed clinical examination, followed by targeted instrumental and specialist investigations when indicated, allows clinicians to define a child's "drooling phenotype", assess aspiration risk, and tailor management according to individual needs and priorities.

Although current evidence is limited, the proposed algorithm balances clinical prudence with resource use, aiming to timely detect aspiration and other complications with the minimum possible risk. Given the heterogeneity of causes, severity, and impact, *shared decision-making with families*, regular follow-up, and periodic re-evaluation are essential. Further research is needed to standardise assessment protocols, validate outcome measures, and define long-term trajectories and optimal interventions.

References

1. Melo B, Araújo R, Azevedo MJ, Amorim R, Palhau L. Management of sialorrhoea in children. Pediatr Oncall. 2021;18(3):71–6.
2. Little SA, Kubba H, Hussain SSM. An evidence-based approach to the child who drools saliva. Clin Otolaryngol. 2009;34:236–9.
3. Saniasiaya J, van der Meer G, Toll EC. Drooling in developmentally normal children: a review. J Laryngol Otol. 2024;138(11):1061–4.
4. Dias BLS, Fernandes AR, Maia Filho HS. Sialorrhea in children with cerebral palsy. J Pediatr (Rio J). 2016;92(6):549–58.
5. Speyer R, Cordier R, et al. Prevalence of drooling, swallowing, and feeding problems in people with cerebral palsy: a systematic review. Dev Med Child Neurol. 2019;61(11):1249–58.
6. Gandhi K, Strychowsky J, Chen B. Pediatric sialorrhea (drooling). CMAJ. 2024;13(196):E624.
7. Sialorrhoea (drooling) in children – clinical guideline 1187. www.rightdecisions.scot.nhs.uk.
8. Sforza E, Onesimo R, Leoni C, Giorgio V, Proli F, Notaro F, Kuczynska EM, Cerchiari A, Selicorni A, Rigante D, Zampino G. Drooling outcome measures in paediatric disability: a systematic review. Eur J Pediatr. 2022;181(7):2575–92.
9. Saliva control in children – an information guide for families and children. www.rch.org.au.
10. Reid.S, Johnson H, Reddihough D. The Drooling Impact Scale: a measure of the impact of drooling in children with developmental disabilities. Dev Med Child Neurol. 2009;52(2):e23–8.

11. Sialorrhea in cerebral palsy. www.aacpdm.org/publications/care-pathways/sialorrhea-in-cerebral-palsy.
12. Haas R, Bailey S. Clinical and instrumental swallowing assessments for dysphagia: rapid review. CADTH Health Technology Review; 2024.
13. Clunie G. Choosing instrumental assessments of swallowing for children. ENT & Audiology News; 2024.
14. Lawlor CM, Choi SS. Videofluoroscopic swallow study and fiberoptic endoscopic evaluation of swallow, which is superior? Laryngoscope. 2023;133(10):2445–6.
15. Rubasinghe MS, Jayathilake SMSW, Udugama KLLG. Instrumental swallowing assessment in children. ResearchGate Review; 2024.
16. Tutor J. Dysphagia and chronic pulmonary aspiration in children. Pediatr Rev. 2020;41(5):236–44.
17. Abu-Hasan, et al. Salivary amylase level in bronchoalveolar fluid as a marker of chronic pulmonary aspiration in children. Pediatr Allergy Immunol Pulmonol. 2014;27(3):115–9.
18. Suzuki T, Saitou M, Utano Y, Utano K, Niitsuma K. Association between HRCT image findings of aspiration pneumonia and elevated bronchoalveolar lavage amylase and pepsin. Eur Respir J. 2023;62(suppl 67):PA5117.

Intraoral Appliance for Paediatric Salivary Control

4

Lau May Nak

4.1 Introduction

Drooling represents a common and often persistent challenge among children with compromised oral-motor control. It is most frequently associated with reduced orofacial muscle tone, often referred to clinically as orofacial hypotonia, as well as impaired swallowing coordination or broader neurological dysfunction such as cerebral palsy, genetic syndromes, neurodevelopmental delay, and neuromuscular disorders [4, 11]. Orofacial hypotonia contributes substantially to drooling by affecting lip seal, tongue stability, and jaw posture, which in turn result in an open-mouth habit, anterior tongue thrust, delayed swallow initiation, and reduced spontaneous swallowing frequency.

Beyond social and hygienic difficulties, including perioral skin irritation, the need for frequent bib or clothing changes, and feeding-related stress, drooling can pose important medical complications. These include chronic perioral dermatitis, dehydration, poor weight gain, recurrent respiratory infections, and aspiration of saliva, which may progress to aspiration pneumonia or, in severe cases, become life-threatening [11, 22]. Thus, the management of drooling extends beyond quality-of-life concerns to become a core component of safeguarding the child's general health and preventing long-term morbidity.

L. M. Nak (✉)
Department of Orthodontics, Paediatric and Special Care Dentistry, Faculty of Dentistry, Universiti Malaya, Kuala Lumpur, Malaysia
e-mail: minalau@um.edu.my

J. Saniasiaya (ed.), *An Overview of Drooling in Children*,
https://doi.org/10.1007/978-981-92-1850-9_4

A range of therapeutic approaches has been proposed to address these functional impairments, including oral-motor therapy, behavioural interventions, pharmacological treatment, and surgical procedures. Within the conservative spectrum, the Castillo Morales appliance, a palatal plate developed as part of the Castillo Morales orofacial regulation therapy concept, has gained attention for its potential to improve oral awareness, promote more appropriate tongue posture, and facilitate more efficient swallowing. Evidence, although limited by small sample sizes, heterogeneity, and an overall low level of certainty, suggests that palatal plates such as the Castillo Morales appliance may reduce drooling severity, increase swallowing frequency, and enhance lip closure in appropriately selected children [8, 14, 18, 21, 23]. This chapter reviews the theoretical background, design principles, clinical application, and current evidence base for the Castillo Morales appliance and highlights practical and interdisciplinary considerations relevant to paediatric drooling management.

4.2 Historical Background and Theoretical Foundations

The Castillo Morales concept originates from the work of Argentine physician Dr. Rodolfo Castillo Morales, whose approach was grounded in neurodevelopmental principles, sensory-motor regulation, and the importance of postural control in facilitating functional movement patterns.

Orofacial regulation therapy (ORT), a core component of this method, emphasises the role of targeted sensory input to the lips, cheeks, tongue, and palate in eliciting improved neuromuscular activation and functional oral movements [5, 6]. The Castillo Morales appliance was subsequently developed to provide structured, repeatable intraoral stimulation that complements the manual techniques delivered by physiotherapists and speech-language therapists. In practice, the palatal plate may be used within therapy sessions to reinforce guided oral-motor activities, or worn independently outside therapy as part of a home programme, providing continuous low-effort sensory input throughout daily routines. The appliance is typically worn for several hours a day, except during eating and sleeping [12], thereby delivering sensory stimulation for a far longer duration than is possible with manual therapy alone. By supporting both therapist-directed exercises and daily sensory experience, the appliance contributes to soft-tissue training and the consolidation of more automatic and physiologic oral-motor patterns.

4.3 Design Features of the Castillo Morales Appliance

The Castillo Morales appliance is a removable or fixed intraoral device custom-made for the upper arch or palate. Typical design elements include a stimulating button, textured sensor zones, and additional components to engage the lips and cheeks [12].

4.3.1 Removable Appliance

The removable Castillo Morales appliance is the most widely used design and is constructed in a manner similar to an upper removable orthodontic appliance. It consists of an acrylic baseplate that conforms closely to the maxillary palate, combined with retentive wire clasps that anchor the appliance securely to the teeth when needed. Following the ARAB principle—Active components, Retentive elements, Anchorage, and Baseplate—the device incorporates active features such as a stimulating button and designated sensor zones to enhance oral awareness and promote appropriate tongue posture (Fig. 4.1). This removable design allows for gradual adaptation, easy cleaning, and ease of adjustment as the child grows while still delivering targeted sensory stimulation during wear.

For infants who have not yet erupted their first teeth, an edentulous version of the Castillo Morales appliance can be fabricated (Fig. 4.2). In this fully edentulous stage, retention is often favourable because the acrylic baseplate can extend broadly over the alveolar ridges and conform closely to the palatal anatomy. This adaptation creates a natural suction effect that provide retention for the appliance. Such approaches are well-established in the design of feeding plates and other early orofacial therapy devices for newborns.

A distinct challenge emerges when the first primary teeth begin to erupt. During this transitional phase, the dental arches do not yet provide adequate crown height or undercuts for reliable clasp engagement, and simultaneous eruption in multiple regions complicates stable adaptation of the acrylic baseplate. Even minor adjustments—such as local reduction of the plate around emerging teeth—may compromise suction and retention. While temporary measures such as modified wire extensions, selective baseplate trimming, soft lining materials, or the use of denture adhesive can provide short-term stability, frequent reviews and repeated adjustments are typically required.

To address this difficulty, Hohoff and Ehmer [14] proposed a staged management approach. When isolated teeth erupt, small relief cavities (approximately 1 mm in

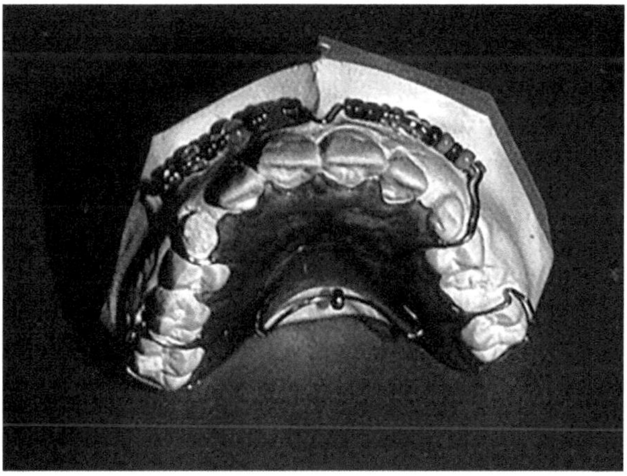

Fig. 4.1 Removable Castillo Morales appliance with movable dorsal bead and labial beads [18]

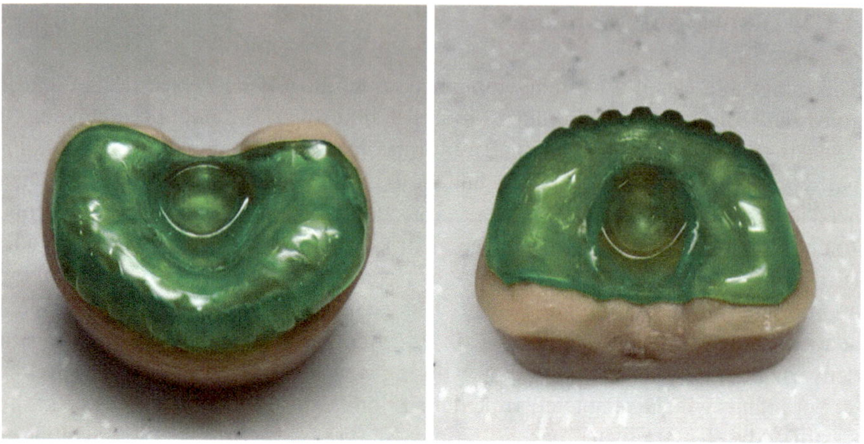

Fig. 4.2 Castillo Morales appliance for infant with dome-shaped stimulating button and textured sensor zone

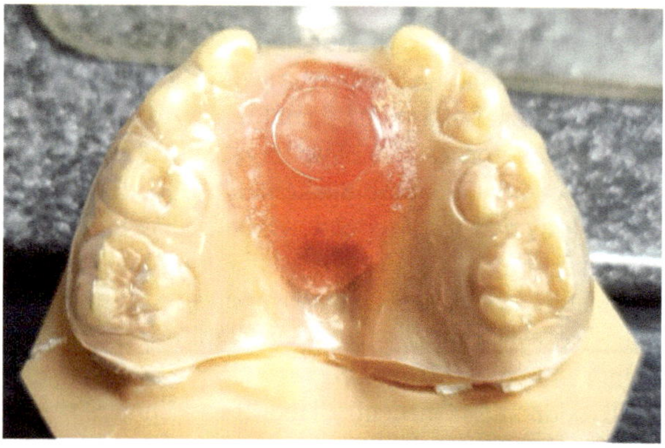

Fig. 4.3 Thermoformed Castillo Morales appliance (Photo courtesy of Mr. Mohamad Najib bin Mohamad Ibrahim)

diameter) may be incorporated into the plate to accommodate the erupting crowns while preserving overall fit. However, the authors noted that extensive or multiple tooth eruptions make reliable adaptation challenging. In such cases, they recommend temporarily interrupting appliance therapy during periods of active eruption. During this interval, alternative orofacial interventions—particularly physiotherapy and speech-language therapy—should be intensified to maintain therapeutic progress. Once the primary dentition is fully erupted and provides sufficient undercuts for mechanical retention, appliance therapy can be resumed as a second treatment stage using conventional clasp-retained designs.

After full eruption of the primary or permanent teeth, appliance retention becomes more predictable. Adequate clinical crown height allows for the use of standard retentive components such as Adams clasps or ball clasps, restoring the stability needed for consistent therapeutic wear. In addition to conventional acrylic designs, a variant fabricated using thermoformed materials can also be employed (Fig. 4.3).

While the removable design offers advantages in gradual adaptation, hygiene, and adjustability, it also presents several limitations when compared with a fixed appliance. Its effectiveness is highly dependent on consistent wear, making treatment vulnerable to poor compliance, especially in young children or those with behavioural or sensory challenges. Removable appliances may be lost, removed frequently, or damaged, reducing overall therapeutic benefit. Retention can be compromised in primary or mixed dentitions with limited clasp engagement, and some children may experience transient speech interference or gag sensitivity during adaptation. In contrast, a fixed appliance ensures continuous wear and uninterrupted sensory stimulation, making it particularly beneficial in children who are unable to maintain a removable plate reliably.

4.3.2 Fixed Appliance

In children who are unable to maintain a removable appliance due to behavioural, cognitive, or motor limitations, a fixed version may be considered. This variant is attached to premolar or molar bands or bonded directly to the teeth, ensuring constant wear and continuous sensory stimulation (Fig. 4.4). Although fixed designs are less frequently described in the Castillo Morales-specific literature, their use is grounded in the same therapeutic principles as the removable variant. However, fixed appliances may complicate oral hygiene maintenance and increase plaque accumulation, thereby elevating the risk of enamel demineralisation, white spot lesions, dental caries, and gingival inflammation if oral hygiene is inadequate.

4.3.3 Selection Considerations

The decision between fixed and removable designs depends on the child's age, level of cooperation, oral-motor function, and caregiver ability to support daily wear and

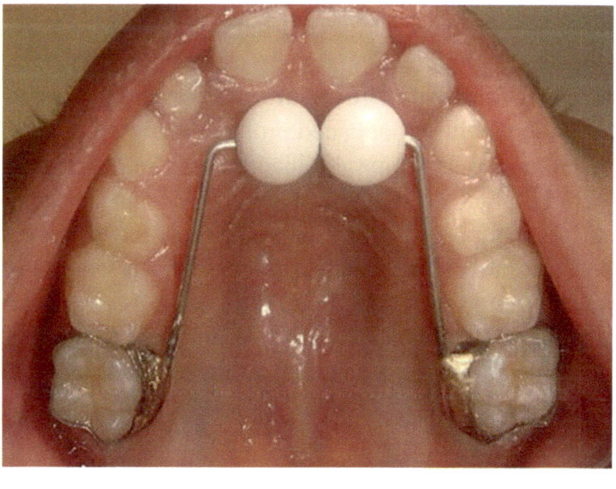

Fig. 4.4 Fixed Castillo Morales appliance [9]

hygiene. Removable plates are preferred when compliance is achievable, whereas fixed appliances may be advantageous when continuous stimulation is required or when repeated loss or removal limits therapeutic benefit. Compared with other similar intraoral devices used in paediatric care, such as oral screens, which primarily aim to improve lip seal [3], or palatal lift appliances and orthodontic airway plates, which mechanically elevate the soft palate or position the tongue anteriorly to address velopharyngeal insufficiency or airway obstruction respectively [7, 13, 26], the Castillo Morales appliance specifically targets sensory-motor integration rather than structural repositioning.

4.3.4 Active Components

4.3.4.1 Palatal Components

Dome-Shaped Stimulating Button (Fig. 4.2 & Fig. 4.3)

A smooth, dome-shaped acrylic prominence is typically positioned on the anterior palate near the rugae region. Its location may be modified to a mid-palatal or posterior position when stimulation of the mid-tongue or dorsal tongue is required. The button provides targeted tactile input, promoting tongue elevation and facilitating palatal-lingual contact.

Movable Dorsal Bead (Fig. 4.1)

Some designs incorporate a bead mounted on a transverse wire, allowing side-to-side movement. Positioned mid- or posteriorly on the palate, the bead stimulates the dorsal tongue, encourages bilateral tongue coordination, and supports improved tongue-body elevation.

Textured Sensor Zones (Fig. 4.2)

Textured zones—formed by lightly ridged, stippled, or grooved acrylic—are placed anteriorly or laterally to enhance oral sensory awareness. When the child explores these zones with the tongue, tactile feedback is increased, supporting swallowing initiation and more active oral-motor patterns.

4.3.4.2 Vestibular Components for the Lips and Cheeks

In children with pronounced orofacial hypotonia or reduced perioral activity, additional components may be incorporated into the labial or buccal vestibule. These include labial beads (Fig. 4.1), cheek stimulation beads, or modified vestibular shields equipped with raised or textured surfaces (Fig. 4.3). These structures are designed to stimulate the orbicularis oris and buccinator muscles, promoting improved lip seal, cheek tone, and perioral stability during swallowing.

If a single appliance design is insufficient to address all therapeutic needs, two or more plates may be used either alternately or sequentially in stages to target distinct oral-motor goals [12].

4.4 Mechanisms Supporting Saliva Control

The Castillo Morales appliance supports improved saliva control through several complementary mechanisms. Its palatal and vestibular components provide continuous low-threshold sensory input that facilitates coordinated oral-motor behaviour [5, 6].

4.4.1 Enhanced Oral Sensory Awareness

The dome-shaped stimulating button, textured sensor zones, and vestibular sensory elements increase oral sensory input to the tongue, lips, and cheeks. This heightened awareness promotes more organised oral activity, facilitates timely swallow initiation, and supports improved management of saliva.

4.4.2 Improved Tongue Posture and Refined Lingual Motor Patterns

Sustained tongue contact with the anterior, mid-palatal, or posterior stimulating button encourages more physiologic tongue resting posture and improved midline orientation of the tongue. When a movable bead is present, dynamic interaction supports bilateral coordination, lateralisation, and dorsal tongue elevation. These motor adjustments strengthen intrinsic and extrinsic tongue musculature and reduce maladaptive patterns such as anterior tongue thrust.

4.4.3 Improved Mandibular Positioning and Lip Seal

The acrylic baseplate provides proprioceptive input that promotes a more stable mandibular rest posture, reducing habitual open-mouth posture. Improved jaw stability facilitates lip approximation, which is essential for containing saliva and reducing anterior escape.

4.4.4 Activation of Perioral Musculature (Lips and Cheeks)

Vestibular components such as labial beads, buccal stimulation beads, or modified vestibular shields deliver gentle sensory pressure to the orbicularis oris and buccinator muscles. This supports lip competence, improved cheek tone, and enhanced perioral stability during swallowing.

4.4.5 Consolidation of Motor Learning and Swallowing Automaticity

Repeated exposure to palatal and perioral sensory-motor experiences during appliance wear reinforces the neuromuscular pathways necessary for coordinated swallowing. Over time, these experiences support automaticity and generalisation of improved swallowing patterns, contributing to long-term reductions in drooling.

4.5 Evidence for the Castillo Morales Appliance

Evidence supporting the use of the Castillo Morales appliance is drawn mostly from case report, case series, retrospective, and observational studies. While findings consistently suggest potential benefit in improving oral-motor function and reducing drooling, the overall level of evidence remains low, with significant methodological limitations across studies.

4.5.1 Short-Term Effects

Short-term evaluations consistently report improvements in oral-motor posture and function during active treatment. Hohoff and Ehmer [14] documented significant increases in mouth closure, reductions in tongue protrusion, and improved lip-tongue relationships after approximately 4 months of therapy. Parents likewise observed better mouth and tongue positioning while the plate was worn, suggesting that sensory stimulation and guided tongue positioning may produce early functional gains.

Additional support is provided by a retrospective review of 53 children treated for problematic drooling, in which 72% showed overall improvement and 63% experienced statistically significant reductions in drooling severity and frequency based on the Thomas-Stonell and Greenberg scale [18]. These outcomes were achieved in children selected specifically for their ability to swallow on command, comply with the palatal plate, and demonstrate sufficient patient and parental motivation. Among this suitable cohort, those who improved were also less likely to require escalation to botulinum toxin injections or surgery, indicating that the appliance can serve as a conservative alternative in appropriately selected candidates.

Case-based evidence further illustrates additional functional gains. In a child with intellectual disability exhibiting mouth breathing, lip incompetence, tongue thrusting, and anterior open bite, therapy with a Castillo Morales appliance was associated with progressive improvements in tongue and lip movements, reduction of the open bite, and concurrent improvement in drooling [23]. Although limited to a single case, this supports the biological plausibility of early functional changes induced by targeted palatal stimulation.

4.5.2 Long-Term Effects

Long-term follow-up studies, though limited, suggest that early improvements may persist beyond the active treatment period. Hohoff and Ehmer [14] reported that many children maintained or further enhanced their gains up to approximately 53 months after treatment. Improvements in mouth closure, intraoral tongue rest posture, and overall orofacial appearance remained evident during follow-up, with parental reports reflecting sustained functional benefit. These findings indicate that early sensorimotor changes may consolidate into more stable motor patterns over time.

4.5.3 Effects in Children with Down Syndrome

Children with Down syndrome frequently present with hypotonia, open-mouth posture, anterior tongue placement, and difficulties coordinating oral function, making them a prominent population for palatal plate interventions. A systematic review involving approximately 300 children with Down syndrome found consistent improvements in mimetic muscle tone, tongue retraction, and lip closure following therapy based on the Castillo Morales concept [8]. Treatment typically involved appliance use two to three times daily over periods of 12–48 months, often combined with structured orofacial physiotherapy or speech-language therapy. The most favourable outcomes were reported when therapy commenced before 3 months of age.

Although encouraging, these findings arise from studies with heterogeneous protocols, small samples, and largely non-standardised clinical assessments [1, 24]. A more recent review similarly concluded that studies involving children with Down syndrome and cerebral palsy dominate the evidence base, while research in non-syndromic populations remains sparse. The overall level of evidence was rated as very low, and the authors emphasised the need for well-designed randomised controlled trials with larger sample sizes and more consistent outcome measures [21]. These limitations underscore that, while trends across studies indicate potential benefit, the certainty of evidence remains low and further robust research is required.

4.6 Clinical Procedures for Using the Appliance

Candidate suitability for the Castillo Morales appliance is determined by a combination of characteristic orofacial features originally described in the Castillo Morales concept and practical clinical considerations identified in contemporary clinical practice. According to these foundational indications, appropriate candidates typically present with a broad, hypotonic tongue that frequently adopts an interdental or interlabial position, a tongue showing diastasis with associated protrusion, or an inactive, hypotonic upper lip with narrowed lateral segments. These features reflect reduced oral-motor control and compromised oral posture, which are central therapeutic targets of the appliance [5].

In addition to these structural and functional characteristics, behavioural and physiological readiness is essential. Clinical experience and contemporary studies emphasise that suitable candidates should be able to initiate a swallow when prompted, tolerate the presence of an intraoral device, and have caregivers who are motivated and able to support consistent appliance use. Children who are unable to swallow on command, who show pronounced oral defensiveness or marked gagging, or whose families are unable to commit to regular therapy are less likely to benefit [18].

Beyond these formal criteria, practical clinical assessment remains crucial. Children who demonstrate at least intermittent elevation of the tongue towards the palate—either spontaneously or in response to simple stimulation—are more likely to benefit from the sensory cues provided by the appliance. During examination, the clinician observes the tongue at rest, its ability to move towards the rugae region, and the child's overall tolerance of gentle intraoral contact. Children who accept brief palatal or vestibular touch without excessive distress generally adapt well, whereas those with severe oral hypersensitivity, unstable gag reflexes, or pronounced oral aversion may require preparatory oral-motor or sensory regulation therapy before an intraoral appliance can be considered.

In summary, ideal candidates are those who display the characteristic orofacial features described in the Castillo Morales framework, demonstrate functional readiness such as the ability to swallow on command, tolerate brief intraoral stimulation, and have caregivers who can support consistent use. Conversely, children with minimal tongue-palate contact, significant oral defensiveness, medical contraindications, or insufficient caregiver engagement are less suitable for appliance therapy at that stage.

Once the child is deemed suitable for Castillo Morales appliance therapy, the clinical workflow proceeds through impression-taking or digital scanning, appliance design selection, laboratory fabrication, clinical fitting, and, for removable designs, a structured adaptation schedule, followed by regular reviews for adjustment and monitoring.

For the removable Castillo Morales appliance, a structured adaptation schedule is typically introduced after fitting to support acceptance and ensure comfortable wear. Instead of beginning with full recommended wear duration, the appliance is introduced using a graded approach, starting with very short, supervised periods and gradually increasing wear time over the course of several days or weeks as tolerance improves. This progressive introduction promotes desensitisation, reduces the likelihood of gagging or behavioural rejection, and allows caregivers to observe the child's comfort, swallowing pattern, and changes in drooling frequency. Although the theoretical rationale for graded adaptation is well-established in orofacial regulation therapy and paediatric oral-motor intervention literature, direct evidence demonstrating its superiority over immediate full-time wear remains limited.

For fixed Castillo Morales appliance, the workflow differs from removable designs. Because fixed devices do not rely on voluntary compliance, the clinician typically conducts an in-mouth trial by placing the appliance in its intended position without cement to evaluate the child's tolerance. Acceptable tolerance refers to the child's ability to manage the presence of the appliance without excessive gagging, distress, sudden withdrawal, or defensive behaviour. If tolerated, the fixed appliance can be cemented or bonded during the same visit. Caregivers should be counselled about expected changes in oral sensation, a possible short-term increase in salivary flow, and the need for meticulous oral hygiene to maintain mucosal integrity.

In some children, especially those with significant behavioural challenges, sensory defensiveness, or limited cooperation, an in-mouth trial may not be feasible for either removable or fixed appliances. When a fixed appliance is strongly indicated but placement cannot be attempted awake, cementation under sedation may be considered. This allows safe delivery of the appliance without distress; however, because tolerance cannot be assessed beforehand, early post-placement monitoring is essential.

Regular follow-up appointments, regardless of appliance type, allow the clinician to monitor compliance in the case of removable designs, identify breakages if any, assess drooling severity, evaluate oral-motor changes, adjust stimulating components when required, review mucosal health, and ensure that the appliance remains appropriate as the child grows.

4.7 Interdisciplinary Management

Effective management of drooling in children requires close interdisciplinary collaboration, including paediatric ENT specialists, respiratory physicians, orthodontists, speech-language therapists, and caregivers, among others. The Castillo Morales appliance functions most successfully when integrated within a coordinated multidisciplinary plan.

Paediatric ENT involvement is especially valuable during the initial phase of treatment. Many children experience a transient increase in salivary flow or heightened oral sensory response when first introduced to an intraoral appliance. In such situations, ENT colleagues can help optimise the timing and selection of adjunctive medical therapies, including short-term pharmacological agents or transdermal patches, to support tolerance and reduce excessive drooling during early adaptation. In children who have recently received botulinum toxin injections to the salivary glands, careful coordination of appliance therapy allows both interventions to be timed for maximum therapeutic effect while avoiding overtreatment. Equally important, ENT assessment of airway patency, nasal obstruction, adenoidal hypertrophy, or concomitant respiratory concerns provides critical information that influences appliance design and the child's readiness for intraoral therapy.

Speech-language therapists play an integral role in identifying the specific oral-motor deficits that the appliance should target. Their assessment of tongue posture, lip seal, cheek tone, swallowing pattern, and oral sensory responsiveness guides decisions about the selection and positioning of stimulating elements within the appliance. This collaborative planning ensures that the active components address the child's individual needs, whether the priority is enhancing tongue retraction, improving anterior tongue elevation, supporting lip closure, or increasing intraoral sensory awareness. Ongoing feedback from speech-language therapists also helps refine therapy goals as the child progresses and allows adjustments to be made in appliance wear schedule or component configuration.

The Castillo Morales appliance should not be used in isolation but rather as part of an integrated therapeutic programme. Consistent with the broader literature on palatal plate interventions—particularly in children with Down syndrome—the appliance is most effective when combined with structured orofacial physiotherapy or speech-language therapy. These therapies provide the active oral-motor training and manual stimulation that complement the sensory cues delivered by the appliance, enabling more coordinated tongue movements, improved lip closure, and better swallowing patterns. The synergy between appliance therapy and guided orofacial intervention is therefore essential, as the appliance alone cannot fully address the complex neuromuscular components of drooling. Integrating both approaches ensures that improvements achieved through intraoral stimulation are reinforced through functional training, supporting more stable and meaningful long-term outcomes [8].

Regular communication among members of the multidisciplinary team is essential throughout treatment, as it helps align therapeutic strategies and ensures that the Castillo Morales appliance continues to function as part of a cohesive and well-coordinated management plan. Such interdisciplinary collaboration not only improves clinical outcomes but also supports families by providing a consistent and integrated approach to care. The effectiveness of this model is further enhanced when services are delivered through a one-stop multidisciplinary clinic, which allows coordinated assessment, shared decision-making, and timely adjustment of interventions within a single visit. This structure reduces caregiver burden, strengthens continuity of care, and facilitates more efficient and synergistic teamwork among treating professionals.

4.8 Emerging Directions and Future Work

Digital dentistry is rapidly reshaping the design and fabrication of oral appliances including palatal plates such as the Castillo Morales appliance, offering significant improvements in reproducibility and workflow efficiency. Advances in intraoral scanning, computer-aided design, and both additive and subtractive manufacturing now allow clinicians to produce appliances with greater accuracy and consistency. Recent in vitro work has demonstrated that digitally fabricated palatal plates for newborns and infants meet clinically acceptable accuracy thresholds, with subtractive milling achieving the highest trueness and precision and direct light processing (DLP) at 100 μm providing an effective balance between accuracy and fabrication time [2]. Other studies have similarly shown the feasibility of fully digital workflows for infants with craniofacial anomalies or Down syndrome, with good appliance fit and early functional acceptability [10, 27].

Complementary research on 3D printable materials indicates that emerging printable resins possess mechanical, biological, and processing characteristics suitable for intraoral use, although long-term ageing and biocompatibility require further evaluation. Emerging evidence from related orthodontic applications highlights important variability in the long-term behaviour of 3D-printed resins. A recent 1-year simulated ageing study demonstrated that Ortho Flex (NextDent, Vertex-Dental B.V., Soesterberg, the Netherlands) exhibited the most favourable ageing profile, showing significant increases in flexural strength and hardness after thermocycling and mechanical brushing compared with the other printed material tested [25]. In contrast, findings from a separate comparative study indicated that commonly used 3D-printed resins, including Formlabs Dental LT Clear V2 and NextDent Ortho Flex, were more susceptible to surface degradation, optical deterioration, increased brittleness, and higher water sorption than traditional thermoplastic materials under wet and aged conditions [20]. Together, these results suggest that although 3D printing offers workflow and customisation advantages, material performance remains resin-dependent and sensitive to intraoral ageing, underscoring the need for careful material selection and continued development of more stable and durable printable polymers for long-term intraoral use.

Beyond fabrication and materials, developments in artificial intelligence offer additional opportunities for innovation. Machine learning-based prediction of craniofacial growth has already been demonstrated in several contexts [15, 16, 17, 19, 28], and AI-driven automation is increasingly being used to support orthodontic appliance design. When combined with the established concept of sequential appliance fabrication in clear aligner therapy, these technologies suggest the possibility of future systems capable of generating growth-adaptive series of palatal plates. Such systems could, in principle, use predictive modelling to anticipate palatal development and automate the production of sequential appliances tailored to future growth stages, although this remains an aspirational direction for research rather than a current clinical capability.

Another potential avenue for growth adaptation can be drawn from the split orthodontic airway plate (SOAP) introduced by Stanford, which incorporates a midline expansion screw to accommodate maxillary growth without requiring repeated fabrication of new appliances. This modification of the Tübingen Palatal Plate allows progressive widening as the infant's palate develops, maintaining therapeutic function over longer treatment periods and reducing the need for frequent remakes [7]. A similar concept could, in principle, be translated to future iterations of the Castillo Morales appliance, enabling gradual adjustments to palatal dimensions or stimulating elements as the child grows. Integrating mechanical expanders or digitally predicted growth adjustments may enhance treatment continuity and support more stable long-term outcomes.

Taken together, these technological developments point to several priorities for future research: establishing standardised digital design and manufacturing protocols, validating the long-term biocompatibility and ageing behaviour of printable materials, developing objective and reproducible outcome measures for oral-motor function, and undertaking larger, methodologically robust clinical studies. As digital, AI-assisted, and growth-adaptive workflows continue to mature, they offer the potential not only to enhance the precision and efficiency of palatal plate fabrication but also to generate stronger evidence for their clinical effectiveness. Ultimately, these innovations may expand the therapeutic possibilities of palatal plate interventions and improve the quality and continuity of care for children with oral-motor dysfunction and drooling.

4.9 Conclusion

The Castillo Morales palatal plate provides a non-invasive approach to paediatric drooling management within an interdisciplinary framework. By delivering targeted sensory stimulation and supporting improved oral-motor activation, the appliance can enhance tongue posture, lip seal, and swallowing efficiency in selected children. Observational studies and clinical experience suggest potential short- and long-term benefits, particularly when the appliance is combined with structured orofacial physiotherapy or speech-language therapy. However, the overall level of evidence remains low, and findings should be interpreted cautiously. Future research employing standardised outcome measures, larger and more diverse samples, and well-designed prospective or randomised studies is needed to clarify its effectiveness and define optimal indications. As digital workflows, advanced materials, and growth-adaptive designs continue to evolve, they may further refine the role of the Castillo Morales appliance and expand the therapeutic possibilities for children with drooling and oral-motor dysfunction.

References

1. Anne-Laure B, Davit-Béal T, Lia Yacoub JL, Germa A. Early oral functional therapy in Down syndrome: need for evidence. J Clin Images Med Case Rep. 2023;4(11):2714.
2. Aretxabaleta M, Unkovskiy A, Koos B, Spintzyk S, Xepapadeas AB. Accuracy evaluation of additively and subtractively fabricated palatal plate orthodontic appliances for newborns and infants: an in vitro study. Materials. 2021;14(15):4103.
3. Bengtsson L, Dotevall H, Sjögreen L, Ragnemalm L, Tuomi L. Effects of oral screen exercise on orofacial and pharyngeal activity: an exploratory study using videofluoroscopy and surface electromyography in healthy adults. Clin Exp Dent Res. 2022;8(2):519–28.
4. Blasco PA, Allaire JH. Drooling in the developmentally disabled: management practices and recommendations. Dev Med Child Neurol. 1992;34(10):849–62.
5. Castillo-Morales R, Brondo J. Die orofaziale Regulationstherapie. München: Pflaum Verlag; 1991.
6. Castillo-Morales R, Brondo J, Hoyer H, Limbrock GJ. Treatment of chewing, swallowing and speech defects in handicapped children with Castillo-Morales orofacial regulator therapy: advice for pediatricians and dentists. Zahnärztl Mitt. 1985;75(9):935–42.
7. Choo H, Kim SH, Ahn HW, Poets CF, Chung KR. Split orthodontic airway plate: an innovation to the utilization method of conventional orthodontic airway plate for neonates with Robin sequence. Korean J Orthod. 2022;52(4):308–12.
8. Chouchene F, Masmoudi F, Baaziz A, Maatouk F, Ghedira H. Palatal plate therapy in children with Down syndrome: a systematic review. Int J Dent Oral Sci. 2021;8(11):5076–83.
9. Diwanji A, Jain P, Doshi J, Somani P, Mehta D. Modified bluegrass appliance: a nonpunitive therapy for thumb sucking in pediatric patients—a case report with review of the literature. Case Rep Dent. 2013;2013(1):537120.

10. do Nascimento NF, Warol F, Lima P, Amaral LD, dos Reis DB, Picciani BL. Technical note of a 3D printed stimulating palatal plate prototype for children with trisomy 21. J Clin Exp Dent. 2025;17(2):e136.
11. Erasmus CE, van Hulst K, Rotteveel LJ, Jongerius PH, van den Hoogen FJ, Roeleveld N, et al. Drooling in cerebral palsy: hypersalivation or dysfunctional oral motor control? Dev Med Child Neurol. 2009;51(6):454–9.
12. Fischer-Brandies H, Avalle C, Limbrock GJ. Therapy of orofacial dysfunctions in cerebral palsy according to Castillo-Morales: first results of a new treatment concept. Eur J Orthod. 1987;9(1):139–43.
13. Greene LE, Wilson K, McIntyre G, Wilson J, Mehendale FV. A novel patient-controlled bidirectional palatal lift appliance. Cleft Palate Craniofac J. 2015;52(1):96–101.
14. Hohoff A, Ehmer U. Short-term and long-term results after early treatment with the Castillo Morales stimulating plate: a longitudinal study. J Orofac Orthop. 1999;60(1):2–12.
15. Kaźmierczak S, Juszka Z, Fudalej P, Mańdziuk J. Prediction of facial growth direction with machine learning methods. https://arxiv.org/abs/2106.10464 [Preprint]. 2021.
16. Kim E, Kuroda Y, Soeda Y, Koizumi S, Yamaguchi T. Validation of machine learning models for craniofacial growth prediction. Diagnostics. 2023;13(21):3369.
17. Lyros I, Vastardis H, Tsolakis IA, Kotantoula G, Lykogeorgos T, Tsolakis AI. Growth prediction in orthodontics: a systematic review of past methods up to artificial intelligence. Children. 2025;12(8):1023.
18. Marinone S, Gaynor W, Johnston J, Mahadevan M. Castillo Morales appliance therapy in the treatment of drooling children. Int J Pediatr Otorhinolaryngol. 2017;103:129–32.
19. Myers M, Brown MD, Badirli S, Eckert GJ, Johnson DH, Turkkahraman H. Long-term predictive modelling of the craniofacial complex using machine learning on 2D cephalometric radiographs. Int Dent J. 2025;75(1):236–47.
20. Neoh SP, Khantachawana A, Chintavalakorn R, Santiwong P, Srikhirin T. Comparison of physical, mechanical, and optical properties between thermoplastic materials and 3D-printing resins for orthodontic clear retainers. Am J Orthod Dentofacial Orthop. 2025;167(1):95–109.
21. Pelkonen AM, Närhi L, Häkli S, Raatikainen AM, Pirttiniemi P, Silvola AS. Effectiveness of oral motor appliances on oral motor function and speech in children: a systematic review. Acta Odontol Scand. 2024;82(1):9–17.
22. Reid SM, Johnson HM, Reddihough DS. The drooling impact scale: a measure of the impact of drooling in children with developmental disabilities. Dev Med Child Neurol. 2010;52(2):e23–8.
23. Shin SY, Lee KE, Kim MS, Nam OH, Choi SC, Lee HS. Castillo-Morales appliance therapy in a drooling child with intellectual disability. Int J Disabil Oral Health. 2021;17(1):15–20.
24. Svensson H, Eriksson I. Oral motor therapy with palatal plates in children with Down syndrome–a systematic review [Master's thesis]. Malmö: Malmö University; 2017.
25. Tan ZY, Lau MN, Ahmad Fauzi NA, Radzi Z. Mechanical properties of direct-printed versus thermoformed retainers: a simulated one-year in vitro study [Master's thesis]. Kuala Lumpur: University of Malaya; 2025.
26. Wolfaardt JF, Wilson FB, Rochet A, McPhee L. An appliance-based approach to the management of palatopharyngeal incompetency: a clinical pilot project. J Prosthet Dent. 1993;69(2):186–95.
27. Xepapadeas AB, Weise C, Frank K, Spintzyk S, Poets CF, Wiechers C, et al. Introducing a digital workflow for newborns with craniofacial anomalies: 3D-printed and milled palatal stimulation plates for trisomy 21. BMC Oral Health. 2020;20:20.
28. Zhang JN, Lu HP, Hou J, Wang Q, Yu FY, Zhong C, et al. Deep learning–based prediction of mandibular growth trend in children with anterior crossbite using cephalometric radiographs. BMC Oral Health. 2023;23(1):28.

Behavioural Therapy and Oral Motor Therapy in Managing Drooling in Children

5

Mei Hui Lee and Kah Pheng Oo

5.1 Case History and Parent/Caregiver Interview

The assessment starts with a detailed case history that is collected through structured interviews with family members. This approach will help to investigate possible medical, developmental, and environmental causes of drooling [8].

(a) *Medical history*: a comprehensive and detailed medical history is necessary for the management of saliva control, as it allows the SLT to identify the underlying medical, structural, or neurological factors that may contribute to drooling problems. For children with more than one disability or a complicated one, their medical history often shows that more investigations are needed to understand the child's current medical conditions. These include neurological diagnoses, seizure activity, respiratory status, medications [25] (e.g. benzodiazepines, clobazam), and previous surgical or pharmacological treatments [9, 10, 31].
(b) *Feeding and swallowing history*: feeding information can be obtained from more than one source and in many different ways [2, 20, 55]. Family members may complete the questionnaire before attending the assessment session. During the evaluation session, an SLT can carry out interviews to obtain further information on feeding and swallowing history. A combination of questionnaire and interview is likely to provide the most complete and accurate information on the child [8, 17].

Feeding history includes questions related to:

M. H. Lee
Pusat Perubatan Universiti Malaya, Petaling Jaya, Malaysia
e-mail: mhlee@ummc.edu.my

K. P. Oo (✉)
Child Development Department, Sunway Medical Centre, Petaling Jaya, Malaysia

J. Saniasiaya (ed.), *An Overview of Drooling in Children*,
https://doi.org/10.1007/978-981-92-1850-9_5

(a) *Positioning during feeding*: the alignment and posture of the child's body and head while being fed or self-fed. Proper positioning is important for safe and efficient swallowing as it helps to prevent aspiration [2, 43].
(b) *Duration of feeding*: long feeding time (e.g. over 30 min for a typical meal) can cause fatigue, poor suck/swallow/breathe coordination, or inefficiency in chewing/swallowing. This may lead to reduced food intake, and the child may show frustration [6, 58].
(c) *Interval time between feedings*: the time between feedings helps you figure out when the child is hungry and how much food they can hold.
(d) *Alternative feeding*: a nasogastric (NG) tube, a gastrostomy (G-tube), and total parenteral nutrition (TPN) are some of the alternative feeding methods used to understand a child's nutrition intake and swallowing ability.
(e) *Liquid consistency/food texture*: liquid consistencies (thickened liquids) include level 1 slightly thick, level 2 mildly thick, level 3 moderately thick, and level 4 extremely thick, and food textures (dysphagia diet) include pureed, minced, and moist, or soft and bite-sized [12].
(f) *Respiratory status*: breathing quality and rate during and immediately after feeding. Check whether the child is on oxygen support or non-invasive ventilation (NIV), as these modalities will give information about respiratory effort and overall tolerance [40].
(g) *Signs of distress or behaviour during feeding*: this includes body arching, pushing food away, turning the head to the other side, crying during feeding, showing signs of fear or anxiety, making a facial grimace after swallowing, grabbing away the spoon, and refusing to open the mouth voluntarily. They may also show pleasure feeling during feeding, showing calmness and a happy mood with food [34, 37].
(h) *Sleep patterns*: the amount and quality of sleep, as well as fatigue and alertness, may affect the control of saliva.
(i) *Cognitive and communication status*: intervention may work better if the child can follow basic instruction and is able to have simple communications with family members [24].

(c) *Environmental and behavioural factors*: it is important to identify potential triggers that may increase drooling, and the list includes factors like fatigue, excitement, concentration, or teething [28]. These factors may lead to more noticeable drooling during daytime activities. When removing potential factors, the SLT may ask parents to observe if the child's drooling behaviour changes.

The interview process helps determine whether drooling is primarily motor, sensory, behavioural, or medical. The process also provides a baseline for goal-setting and outcome evaluation [3, 36].

5.2 Oral Motor and Functions Assessment

The oral motor clinical assessment consists of a physical examination, oral structure, and oral motor function assessment.

(a) *Physical Examination*: This is to evaluate the child's muscle tone, basic reflexes, and posture control while they are in a resting posture or moving around. The first step in oral motor therapy is to determine the best posture for stability [2, 43].
(b) *Jaw*: The resting (neutral) position of the jaw is observed to see whether it is protruded or retracted. The assessment of range of motion and symmetry is carried out through imitation tasks, including the action of opening and closing the mouth. The SLT puts gentle downward pressure on the child's jaw while the child keeps their mouth closed to see how strong it is. Significant downward motions can help determine abnormal movements, including jaw thrusts. The SLT will examine the size of the jaw compared to the tongue and the buccal cavity to see if macrognathia or micrognathia is present.
(c) *Lips*: The lips are examined at rest to assess their symmetry. Bilabial closure is evaluated when the child's teeth or gums are in contact, and older children should be capable of sustaining lip closure for up to 5 s at rest. The tone of the top and lower lips is checked separately. It can be high, low, or normal. The child's lip movement is assessed by instructing them to imitate actions such as opening and closing their lips, rounding their lips, and spreading their lips. The SLT evaluates lip strength by applying gentle resistance during these movements. Observations of asymmetry, limited range of motion, or weakness provide important information about oral motor control at the lips.
(d) *Tongue*: The tongue is examined in relation to the size of the oral cavity and mandible to identify the presence of macroglossia or microglossia. Any abnormal involuntary movements, such as fasciculations or tremors, are observed and documented. Tongue range of motion and mobility are assessed by asking the child to perform a series of voluntary tongue movements, including protrusion, retraction, lateralisation, and elevation. These movements are evaluated without compensatory support from the jaw or lips to ensure isolated lingual control. Lingual strength is assessed by instructing the child to press the tongue against the inner cheek, while the SLT applies graded external resistance. The child's ability to produce and maintain force is monitored and documented. The overall look of the tongue is also considered; typically a developing tongue should appear soft, thin, and flat at rest, with a rounded tip and adequate range of movements. Structural differences, including signs of ankyloglossia (tongue-tie), are documented if present.
(e) *Hard Palate*: Assessment of the hard palate is conducted through careful visual observation and gentle touch using a gloved finger or oral tool. The SLT looks at the shape of the palate (such as high-arched, narrow, or flat), its width, symmetry, and overall surface condition. Any unusual features like clefts, ridges,

bony growths, redness, or scarring are noted. The child's comfort and sensory response to touch are also observed. These findings help determine how the palate affects tongue placement, food control, chewing, swallowing, and speech quality [2, 22].

5.3 Oral Sensory Assessment

Currently, there is no standardised assessment designed specifically to evaluate oral sensory processing in children with drooling issues. Therefore, drooling assessment will use the standardised sensory questionnaires combined with structured clinical observation of the oral sensory responses during feeding and oral motor examination [2].

Standardised sensory questionnaires provide valuable insight into the child's sensory responses across settings. These questionnaires are not limited to oral functions; they also help to identify sensory processing patterns that may affect feeding, including responses to tactile, auditory, visual, and olfactory stimuli. Results from these questionnaires should be interpreted in conjunction with clinical observations and feeding performance.

Direct observation of the child during feeding is an important component of an oral sensory assessment. The SLT evaluates the child's acceptance of food presentation, reactions to tactile stimuli on the lips and face, tolerance of utensils, and responses to variation of texture, taste, and temperature [38]. Behavioural indicators such as refusal of food, gagging during feeding, prolonged holding of food in the mouth, spitting out mixed textures, or better intake during distraction provide important clues related to sensory modulation [7].

Children with sensory-based oral feeding difficulties usually show strong preferences and avoidance behaviours towards oral input. They may prefer a specific nipple type or flow rate and can experience nipple confusion when changes are introduced. Feeding may be easier when the child is sleepy or just waking, especially during night-time feeds. These children may frequently prefer non-nutritive sucking (e.g. thumb, finger, or pacifier) but show discomfort when others touch their mouth or tongue. They often prefer liquids, especially water, and may gag easily, particularly with solid foods or when a spoon touches the lips. Some children chew on solid foods but keep them in the mouth to avoid swallowing or to separate and spit out pieces of mixed-texture foods. When they are distracted, they may be able to handle and swallow a wider range of food textures [20].

In contrast, children with oral motor-based feeding difficulties mostly struggle with the coordination, strength, and timing of oral movements that are required for efficient feeding. These children may display sucking difficulties across all nipple types and have difficulty adapting to changes in flow rates [18]. Feeding is usually most successful when the child is in a calm, quiet-alert state. Unlike sensory-based issues, these children often tolerate oral touch and allow another person's finger in the mouth for non-nutritive sucking. They may manage pureed or textured foods better than thin liquids but show difficulties with chewing and bolus control. Gagging is less frequent and typically occurs only when the swallow is delayed or when aspiration is present. Mixed food textures are always hard to deal with, and feeding problems usually stay the same, but they can get worse when the child is distracted [20].

Oral sensory dysfunction may present as either hypersensitivity or hyposensitivity, both of which can significantly impact feeding and saliva management. Oral hypersensitivity, characterised by an excessive or overreactive response, may occur in reaction to tactile input during oral care or oral play or following exposure to specific tastes or textures [55]. These children frequently demonstrate gagging, vomiting, or strong behavioural resistance to continuous oral stimulation. Over time, feeding repertoires may become restricted and selective, only allowing foods that meet related sensory criteria for shape, taste, texture, visual appearance, and temperature. Children demonstrating strong responses to oral sensory input often have underlying central nervous system involvement and may show sensitive responses to taste, temperature, and touch in and around the oral area. These responses may indicate increased oral hypertonicity or abnormal oral motor movements, further interfering with feeding efficiency [2].

In contrast, oral hyposensitivity shows an underresponsive sensory pattern and may be observed when a child is not aware of food residue in the oral cavity, diminished flavour perception, or reduced awareness of the amount of food placed intraorally [55]. Children with fewer responses to oral sensory input may show reduced sensitivity to taste, temperature, and the proprioceptive input related to chewing and sucking. Consequently, they may seek increased oral sensory input by preferring strong flavours, crunchy textures, or extreme temperatures; they may also display behaviours such as overstuffing the mouth or persistent drooling [2]. Inadequate sensory feedback can affect the development of efficient sucking and chewing skills, as the child does not receive sufficient sensory information to support the refinement and coordination of oral motor movements.

Oral sensory problems can significantly influence the presence and severity of drooling. Sensory deficit or inadequate sensory awareness of the presence of saliva loss may contribute to drooling [54]. However, motor-based causes must always be considered and not overlooked. Effective drooling control depends on the child's ability to feel saliva within the oral cavity, exhibit a response to this sensory input, and generate an appropriate and timely motor response, such as lip closure, tongue movement, and dry swallow initiation. Oral motor and swallowing impairments frequently coexist with abnormal oral sensory functions; some children may demonstrate both sensory and motor problems in varying degrees [2]. Drooling is most often the result of a combined sensory-motor dysfunction rather than a single isolated deficit.

5.4 Swallowing and Feeding Assessment

Drooling and dysphagia frequently co-occur. Drooling should be viewed as one aspect of a spectrum of impairments related to oral motor and oral sensory function that also includes speech problems, feeding difficulties and swallowing dysfunction, and aspiration [54]. Therefore, when a child presents with drooling, the SLT also performs a clinical swallowing assessment to evaluate swallowing and feeding function.

5.4.1 Bottle Feeding

During the bottle-feeding assessment, both nutritive and non-nutritive sucking are systematically evaluated. The types of bottle and nipple, liquid consistency, and nipple flow are often evaluated. The child's positioning, suckle initiation, and presence of any suckle lag are also documented. The strength of the tongue seal is tested on babies 0–6 months old, and the strength of the lip seal is tested on children 6 months and older. The SLT distinguishes between suckle and sucking patterns by monitoring mandibular excursion and coordination. The suck-to-swallow ratio is compared at the beginning and the end of feeding to identify fatigued muscles, and the length of burst cycles and total feeding duration are documented to assess endurance.

5.4.2 Spoon Feeding

Spoon feeding assessment examines anticipatory skills such as opening the mouth before the spoon approaches it, the jaw adjusting to receive food, and the coordinated movements of the lips, tongue, and cheeks. The SLT also observes how effectively the child can clear the food from the spoon.

5.4.3 Cup Drinking

The cup drinking assessment looks into the movements of the lips, cheeks, and tongue, along with the stability of the jaw. Observations include whether the child bites the cup, how well the child can keep the liquid within the oral cavity, and any spillage during drinking.

5.4.4 Straw Drinking

Straw drinking requires the functions of lip, tongue, and cheek movements and the child's ability to control spillage. Liquid texture or consistency helps to assess the child's sucking strength. The child's ability to control the volume of liquid taken per sip is documented.

5.4.5 Chewing Soft Solids

When assessing soft solid foods, the SLT observes the transition from anterior munching patterns with straight up-and-down jaw movements to diagonal munching patterns that move the jaw from side to side. These movements help the development of mature rotary chewing patterns. The assessment includes observation of bite force and chewing efficiency, lip closure, and coordinated movements of the lips, tongue, cheeks, and jaw.

5.4.6 Chewing Hard Solids

Assessment of hard solid foods focuses on the child's tongue lateralization, including the ability to move food from midline to sides, side to midline, and side to side. The observation also includes the coordination of lip, tongue, cheek, and jaw, along with the maturation of rotary chewing patterns and the child's ability to manage bolus safely and efficiently.

5.5 Phases of Swallow

Swallowing is a complicated process that happens in four steps: the oral preparatory phase, the oral phase, the pharyngeal phase, and the oesophageal phase. These four steps include combining voluntary and involuntary muscle movements, sensory input, and neural control to move food from the mouth to the stomach in a safe and effective way. Impairment at any stage may disrupt bolus control, airway protection, and efficient bolus transport.

The oral preparatory phase and oral phase are voluntary control movements, whereas the pharyngeal phase and oesophageal phase are involuntary control.

The oral preparatory phase begins when food or liquid is introduced into the oral cavity. During this voluntary phase, food is chewed, mixed with saliva, and formed into a cohesive bolus in preparation for transfer to the pharynx. This process requires coordinated movements of the lips, cheeks, tongue, and jaw to contain and manipulate the bolus while preventing premature spillage into the pharynx. Difficulties during this phase may present as bolus loss from the mouth, pooling of food or saliva in the anterior sulci, reduced tongue mobility for bolus formation, and inefficient or reduced chewing.

The oral phase follows and involves the voluntary transport of the prepared bolus from the oral cavity to the oropharynx. This is achieved through an anterior-to-posterior movement of the tongue against the hard palate, accompanied by elevation of the soft palate to seal off the nasopharynx and prevent nasal regurgitation. Impairments in the oral phase may be observed as pooling of food in the lateral sulci, expulsion of food from the mouth, reduced bolus formation, delayed initiation of the swallow, and piecemeal deglutition.

The pharyngeal phase is triggered when the bolus passes the anterior tonsillar pillars and enters the pharynx. This phase is quick and automatic, and it usually lasts about 1 s. During this phase, the soft palate elevates, respiration temporarily ceases, the hyoid and larynx elevate and move anteriorly, and the vocal folds adduct to protect the airway. The pharyngeal constrictor muscles work together to create a peristaltic stripping wave that pushes the bolus towards the upper esophageal sphincter (UES). The UES then relaxes for a short time to let the bolus pass. Signs of pharyngeal phase impairment include reduced laryngeal elevation and anterior movement, gurgly or wet voice quality, and choking or coughing before, during, or after swallowing.

The oesophageal phase is entirely involuntary and begins once the bolus passes through the UES into the oesophagus. During this phase, the bolus is transported to the stomach via coordinated peristaltic waves regulated by the autonomic nervous system. Following bolus passage, the UES closes to prevent retrograde flow, while the lower oesophageal sphincter (LES) relaxes to permit entry of the bolus into the stomach. Oesophageal phase dysfunction may be indicated by complaints of food sticking in the chest or throat, chest discomfort during meals, regurgitation or vomiting of undigested food, a sensation of food or liquid progressively accumulating as the meal continues, and postprandial or nocturnal coughing, particularly in the supine position [35].

The clinical signs and symptoms of dysphagia vary according to the swallowing phase, including the oral phase preparatory phase, oral phase, pharyngeal phase, and oesophageal phase, as summarised in Table 5.1.

Impairments in any phase of swallowing can significantly affect an individual's ability to manage and swallow saliva. When swallowing function is compromised, the frequency of spontaneous saliva swallows is often reduced, and the strength, timing, and coordination of the muscles responsible for saliva clearance are diminished. Saliva accumulates in the oral cavity and may spill either anteriorly or posteriorly, resulting in drooling. Therefore, effective swallowing function plays a crucial role in saliva management, and drooling is frequently a manifestation of underlying oropharyngeal swallowing dysfunction rather than excessive saliva production.

Table 5.1 Clinical signs and symptoms of dysphagia according to swallowing phase

Phase of swallow	Signs and symptoms
Oral preparatory	Bolus spills out of the mouth Pooling in anterior sulci Reduced tongue movement to form bolus Reduced chewing
Oral	Pooling in lateral sulci Food is expelled from the mouth Reduced bolus formation Delayed swallow Piecemeal deglutition
Pharyngeal	Reduced laryngeal excursion and anterior movement Gurgly voice quality Choking or coughing before, during, or after swallowing
Esophageal	Complain about food getting stuck Chest pain with eating Vomiting of undigested food A sensation of gradual filling up of food and liquid as a meal progresses Postprandial and/or nocturnal (supine) coughing

Reference: Arvedson et al. [2], pp. 318–321, Ongkasuwan and Chiou [35], pp. 215–238

5.6 Standardised and Instrumental Drooling Assessment Tools

Assessment tools for drooling can be broadly classified as subjective (perceptual, questionnaire-based) and objective (quantitative, observational, or physiological) measures. Evidence supports combining both to achieve a holistic view [59].

5.6.1 Drooling Severity and Frequency Scale (DSFS)

Developed by Thomas-Stonell and Greenberg [51], the DSFS is one of the most widely used clinical measures. It comprises two subscales:

- Severity (1–5): ranging from 1 = dry to 5 = profuse drooling where clothing and objects become wet
- Frequency (1–4): 1 = never, 2 = occasional, 3 = frequent, 4 = constant

The DSFS is simple, reliable, and sensitive to change following intervention [31, 46]. Its ordinal format makes it useful for monitoring changes over time. However, the results depend on the observer's judgement and may vary between different raters. For younger children, parental reports offer valuable additional perspectives.

5.6.2 Drooling Impact Scale (DIS)

The DIS is a 10-item parent questionnaire evaluating how drooling affects the child's health, comfort, and family life [46]. Each item is rated on a scale from 1 ("not at all") to 10 ("constant"), covering domains such as the frequency of bib changes, skin irritation, odour, and social embarrassment. The total score (10–100) shows the overall effect, and a drop of more than 10 points means that there has been a clinically significant improvement [39]. The DIS demonstrates excellent reliability (ICC = 0.95) and strong construct validity, correlating with caregiver global ratings of change. It is beneficial for evaluating quality-of-life outcomes both before and after intervention.

5.6.3 Drooling Quotient (DQ)

The DQ is a semi-quantitative observational method that is thought to be one of the most objective ways to measure how often someone drools [14, 30]. During a 5–10-min observation, the observer records the presence of new saliva beyond the lip margin every 15 s. The number of intervals showing drooling is divided by the total number of intervals, yielding a percentage score. A 50% decrease in DQ is typically regarded as clinically significant [14]. DQ assessment can be performed at rest (DQ-rest) or during activity (DQ-activity), indicating both passive and task-related saliva regulation. Although it demonstrates strong reliability (ICC > 0.86), the measure requires trained observers and may not represent day-to-day variability.

5.6.4 Drooling Infants and Preschoolers Scale (DRIPS)

The DRIPS [53] provides developmental benchmarks for saliva control in children aged 0–4 years. It rates drooling frequency across everyday contexts such as feeding, play, sleep, and babbling. Using context-based frequency ratings and DRIPS percentile charts, the SLT can compare a child's performance with age norms: scores at or above the 85th percentile signal risk, while those at or above the 97th percentile indicate pathological drooling. The DRIPS is useful for early identification and tracking of saliva control milestones, especially in children with developmental delays.

5.6.5 Visual Analogue Scale (VAS)

The VAS is a simple tool where caregivers rate drooling severity on a 0–100 continuum, where 0 indicates no drooling and 100 signifies the most severe level. It provides a subjective estimate of severity and can complement other assessments by capturing caregiver perceptions of change. However, its interpretability varies between respondents [46].

5.6.6 Instrumental Assessments: VFSS and FEES

Videofluoroscopic Swallow Study (VFSS) and Fiberoptic Endoscopic Evaluation of Swallowing (FEES) offer valuable information regarding drooling pathophysiology. VFSS visualises oral transit and pharyngeal clearance to identify whether saliva is safely managed or aspirated [26]. FEES enables the direct visualisation of laryngeal pooling, penetration, or the silent aspiration of secretions. The SLT uses these tools when posterior drooling or respiratory complications are suspected. The SLT's role includes identifying suitable candidates, selecting the right measures, interpreting results, and integrating findings with behavioural assessments, which are all essential for the evaluation process.

5.7 Drooling Management

From an SLT's perspective, salivary management in the paediatric population involves the use of behavioural and oral motor therapy. These conservative methods are often the first step in treatment, especially for young patients who may not be ready for more invasive treatments yet. The goal of both behavioural and oral motor techniques is to help the child develop better sensory awareness, swallow more frequently, and move their oral muscles (jaw, lip, and tongue) in a coordinated manner so that they can control their saliva [41].

A behavioural intervention for saliva management in children is a non-invasive approach that focuses on teaching the child conscious control and awareness over their salivary and oral movements. It is based on the idea that drooling, especially in children with neurodisabilities (like cerebral palsy or intellectual disability), is often due to an impaired ability to recognise wetness, swallow, or keep their mouth closed, rather than an overproduction of saliva.

5.7.1 Behavioural and Oral Motor Interventions for Drooling

Behavioural and oral motor interventions are highly personalised and generally involve a multidisciplinary team, including SLTs, occupational therapists, and physical therapists [4, 52]. The primary goal of behavioural intervention is not to stop saliva production but to increase the awareness and frequency of swallowing and improve oral motor competence to contain saliva within the oral cavit [42, 48].

1. *Body Posture*

   Stability within the body facilitates mobility in the oral cavity [45]. Maintaining optimal body posture is essential for ensuring stability and facilitating independent motions of the jaw, lips, and tongue.
   (a) A stable posture helps keep the pelvis, knees, ankles, and chin at a 90-degree angle.
   (b) It is important to have both feet on the ground to ensure postural stability.
   (c) For children who are unable to get adequate posture stability, it is recommended to consult a physiotherapist to assist in establishing and maintaining optimal body posture to reduce or prevent drooling.
   (d) Putting a slip-resistant pad on a seat would stop the chair from moving.
2. *Sensory Awareness and Biofeedback*

   Children who experience drooling are often unaware of the saliva escaping from their mouths. Cueing techniques are designed to increase awareness of drooling episodes and promote prompted swallowing or wiping actions [21]. The SLT will consider the child's age, cognitive ability, and sensory profile to choose the most appropriate method to tailor their needs. These may include the following:
   (a) Verbal prompts: use keywords or reminders, such as "swallow" and "close your mouth" [11].
   (b) Gestural prompts: using hand gestures or gentle tapping on the chin to signal the presence of saliva. The child may use a wristband or handkerchief to dab on the chin [29].
   (c) Auditory [27] or electrical devices, such as the Accularm, which generate timed auditory signals to facilitate saliva swallowing [9]. Devices such as Swallow Prompt used timed vibrations or auditory signals to encourage users to swallow before saliva leaves their lips. These devices are user-friendly and widely available from therapy suppliers.

(d) Reinforcement: This approach uses positive reinforcement to establish a connection between desirable behaviour, such as having a dry mouth and voluntarily swallowing and rewards (e.g. verbal praise, tokens, and preferred activities). This is to promote oral dryness and increase self-awareness during the daytime.
(e) Thermal/taste stimulation: Application of cold or sour stimuli, such as a frozen swab or a small amount of lemon juice, can temporarily increase sensory perception and improve saliva awareness, thereby eliciting a more reflexive swallow. The SLT will need to be aware of the potential allergy or oral sensitivity when choosing the correct stimuli.
(f) Sensory stimulation through texture and taste: Incorporating foods or objects with different textures, temperatures, and flavours to improve oral exploration and sensory perception [57].

3. Oral Motor Exercises and Training

   Oral motor therapy consists of specific exercises designed to improve the strength, mobility, and coordination of the muscles associated with eating, speaking, and saliva management.

   1. *Facial Area*

      These exercises aim to improve awareness, tone, and movement in the facial muscles.

      (a) *Facial massage*: This technique is used to increase sensory awareness, decrease hypersensitivity, and relax or stimulate facial muscles at cheek and masseter areas [5, 29, 32].
      (b) *Vibrator*: Devices such as the Z-Vibe provide tactile and proprioceptive input to the face, lips, or oral cavity, thereby increasing sensory awareness and muscle tone. Standard protocols involve 10–15-min sessions with Z-Vibe pulses at 80–100 Hz, applying the device for 2–3 s at each target area [19, 46].
      (c) *Facial expression*: practicing different expressions, such as "happy", "sad", or "surprised", aims to improve range of motion and control of facial muscles, which are important for articulation and non-verbal communication [33].
      (d) *Brushing and icing*: Gentle brushing or the application of cold stimuli (e.g. ice sticks) across the lips, cheeks, and chin to increase oral awareness and trigger swallowing reflexes [15, 19].
      (e) *The blowfish*: The child is instructed to inflate their cheeks with air and maintain the air in the oral cavity (ensuring no air escapes). The therapist then gently taps the cheeks to assess the child's ability to maintain the seal.

      Examples of facial exercises targeting facial muscle activation and sensory stimulation, with step-by-step instructions for implementation during therapy or home practice, are presented in Table 5.2.

Table 5.2 Facial exercises for facial muscle activation and sensory stimulation

Exercise sheet (facial area)
(a) Facial massage: I. Cheeks: Place fingertips on the cheek area (between the jawline and cheekbone) Use gentle circular motions, moving clockwise for 3–5 s and gradually increasing the duration Repeat counterclockwise for another 3–5 s (slowly increase the duration) Apply light to moderate pressure, depending on the child's tolerance Perform on both sides II. Masseter: Identify the masseter by asking the child to clench; look for the muscle bulges at the jaw corner Apply gentle and small circular motions, and massage the muscle for 3–5 s (slowly increase the duration) Stroke gently downward along the jawline to encourage relaxation Perform the massage on both sides III. Around the mouth (perioral area) Apply gentle, small circular motions above the upper lip, around the corners, and below the lower lip Keep pressure light to moderate; sustain the circular motion for 3–5 s (slowly increase the duration)
(b) Vibrator: Use a Z-Vibe or similar vibration tool, starting with low vibration intensity If the child feels anxious, let the child touch and feel the vibration first Turn on the vibrator to the lowest comfortable setting Apply the vibrating tip to the cheek surface and along the border of the lips Use a slow, small circular motion for 3–5 s on each facial area
(c) Facial expression Prepare a few facial expression picture cards, such as "happy", "sad", "surprise", and "angry" Demonstrate the expression and encourage the child to imitate it; for example, show a big smile for the "happy" expression, and maintain the lip retraction for 2–3 s The SLT may use a story or a funny game to encourage the child to perform the expression The SLT may also use a mirror while providing the model so that the child can imitate the expressions
(d) Brushing and icing (sensory stimulation) Sensory stimulation can be given through tactile (brushing) and thermal (icing) forms For brushing, use a soft brush to gently stroke the lips, cheeks, and chin Use small, gentle strokes for 3–4 s Increase the duration and repetitions of the task gradually Perform the stimulation on both sides Repeat the task by using the ice for thermal stimulation
(e) The blowfish exercise (puff cheeks) Ask the child to inhale through the nose and puff out their cheeks Keep the lips sealed tightly Maintain the inflated cheek position for 3–5 s If the child is able to keep the seal, apply a gentle tap on the cheeks to provide resistance

Table 5.3 Jaw exercise program for jaw strength, stability, and graded jaw movement

Exercise sheet (jaw)
(a) Chewy tube or ARK tools Hold the chewy tube with the stem positioned horizontally Place the tip of the chewing tube between the molars on one side of the mouth Prompt the child to "bite down" and "release" Perform the sequence bite → release → bite release for 10 repetitions Encouraging slow and controlled jaw movement, SLT may provide mandible support for better jaw stability The SLT may also use other suitable tools to carry out the steps above
(b) Tug-of-war Use a clean washcloth or a safe chewy tube Place the washcloth or chewy tube between the child's molars on one side Ask the child to bite down firmly on the material Hold the other end and gently pull outward Tell the child, "Don't let me win", and encourage sustained biting down
(c) Vowel singing Sing "Ee-Oo-Ah" in an exaggerated manner *Ee*: Retract lips *Oo*: Round lips *Ah*: Open jaw Moving between these rapidly helps with jaw grading (control of movement)

2. *Jaw*

These techniques focus on improving jaw stability, grading (controlled up-and-down movement), and strength [1, 47].

(a) *Chewy tube*: A durable, non-toxic device used for jaw strengthening, stability, and sensory input through biting and chewing movements. It provides proprioceptive feedback that readies the mouth for speech, helping calm oral seekers and boosting caregiver confidence in its utility.
(b) *ARK tools*: Products (e.g. chew tools, grabbers) designed for oral motor input, providing a safe, resilient, non-food surface for biting and chewing practice to build jaw strength and coordination.
(c) *Crunchy snacking*: Eating crunchy foods (carrots, celery, pretzels, jerky) requires a sustained, rhythmic chew that builds jaw stability [23, 50].
(d) *Tug-of-war*: Use a clean washcloth or a safe chewy tube. Have the child bite down on it with their back teeth (molars) while you gently tug on it. Tell them, "Don't let me win".

Examples of jaw exercises with step-by-step instructions to improve jaw strength, stability, and graded jaw movement are presented in Table 5.3.

3. *Lips*

These exercises enhance lip strength, seal (closure), and mobility for sounds like /p, b, m, w/, as well as maintain oral hygiene and prevent drooling [49].

(a) *Button pulling*: Pull a string through a button and position it just inside the lips. The child will maintain lip closure to hold the button, while the SLT applies a gentle outward pull on the string, thereby strengthening the orbicularis oris muscle.
(b) *Chewy tube*: Can be used to encourage lip rounding and sealing around the stem.
(c) *ARK tools*: Can be used for lip spreading or rounding exercises.
(d) *Tongue depressor*: Holding the tongue depressor horizontally with pursed lips to facilitate lip strength development.
(e) *Blowing*: Activities like blowing bubbles, whistles, or horns, which require a strong and sustained lip seal.
(f) *Lip seal, nasal breathing*: Training the muscles to keep the lips closed (sealed) at rest, promoting breathing through the nose.
(g) *Kissing*: Put lips into kissing (lip pursing) and smiling (lip retraction) movements to strengthen both lip and cheek musculature.
(h) *Sucking*: Using a straw to suck thick liquid, such as a milkshake, or sucking a lollipop to strengthen the cheek and lip muscles.
(i) *Holding a spatula*: Hold a small spatula between the lips, ensuring that the teeth are not used, in a manner similar to the tongue depressor exercise.
(j) *Lip games*:
   - *Raspberry*: A sound made by vibrating the lips (a labial trill), which improves lip closure and breath control.
   - *Humming*: Requires a sustained lip closure (seal) and breath control.

Examples of lip exercises with step-by-step instructions to improve lip strength, closure, and coordination are presented in Table 5.4.

4. *Tongue*

These exercises are crucial for improving the precision and speed of the tongue, which is necessary for producing most speech sounds (articulation) and for moving food during swallowing (bolus manipulation).

(a) *Tongue protrusion*: Sticking your tongue straight out, holding it there, and tracking your progress weekly can make your tongue stronger overall. One way to measure improvement is to time how long the child can maintain the protrusion without tremor. Encourage setting small goals for each week to keep motivation high and celebrate milestones.
(b) *Tongue tip lateralization*: Moving the tongue tip from side to side (e.g. to the corners of the mouth) and cleaning food from the sides of the mouth [13].

Table 5.4 Lip exercises for lip strength, closure, and coordination

Exercise sheet (lips)
(a) Button pulling exercise Attach a short string securely to the button Place the button just inside the child's lips (not between the teeth) Prompt the child to close his or her lips around the button Remind the child not to bite the button Hold the end of the string, and apply a light and steady pulling force outward Remind the child to keep the button in place using lip closure only; try to resist the gentle pull for a few seconds (e.g. 3–5 s) Repeat the exercise for the required number of repetitions
(b) Lip-strengthening exercise Place one end of the tongue depressor between the lips, keeping it horizontal Use lips only to hold it. Avoid using teeth Prompt the child to gently press lips together to secure the tongue depressor Maintain a small, controlled pursed-lip seal The SLT or caregiver may apply mild outward resistance by gently tugging on the free end Remind the child to keep the depressor in place using lip strength Begin with light resistance and increase gradually depending on ability, e.g. hold for 3–5 s, and progress to 5–10 s as strength improves
(c) Blowing exercise Prepare tools based on the child's level and preference; examples of tools are bubbles, whistles, horns, etc Prompt the child to form a tight, rounded lip seal around the blowing tool Ensure the lips (not teeth) are holding the object Prompt the child to take a gentle breath in through the nose Blow steadily and continuously through the tool Maintain the lip seal throughout the entire exhalation Slowly increase the length of blowing from 1–2 s to 3–5 s and more
(d) Lips protrusion and retraction (kissing-smiling) exercise Purse lips forward into an exaggerated kissing shape Hold the position for 2–3 s. Keep the jaw still—Only the lips should move Relax the kiss position Pull lips back into a wide, exaggerated smile Show teeth if possible but maintain a relaxed jaw. Hold it for 2–3 s Move smoothly from kiss → smile → kiss → smile. Repeat the movement Repeat this exercise for 10 cycles, gradually increasing the number of trials as the child becomes more comfortable
(e) Sucking exercise Prepare tools based on the child's level and preference; examples of tools are a straw, a shortened straw (easier suction), a thin narrow straw (increased resistance), a thick consistency liquid (e.g. a smoothie or yogurt drink), a lollipop, etc Prompt the child to place lips around the straw or lollipop Form a tight, complete lip seal; ensure no air leaks from the sides. Avoid biting the straw; just use the lips Inhale gently through the straw, drawing liquid or air in Maintain a steady, continuous suction, e.g. maintain a suction hold on the lollipop for 3 s, and then release

Table 5.5 Tongue exercises for tongue mobility, strength, and coordination

Exercise sheet (tongue)
(a) Tongue protrusion Invite the child to stretch their tongue straight out. An SLT may use a tongue depressor or lollipop as a playful way to encourage the child Hold the position for 3–5 s before relaxing. Slowly increase the duration Repeat the movement 10 times
(b) Tongue tip lateralization Prompt the child to move the tip of the tongue from one corner of the mouth to the other Ensure movements are slow, controlled, and reaching both sides Hold the position for 3–5 s before relaxing. Slowly increase the duration Repeat the movement 10 times
(c) Tongue tip elevation Prompt the child to lift the tip of their tongue towards the alveolar ridge (behind the upper teeth) Elevate the tongue tip and hold for 3–5 s before relaxing Repeat the movement 10 times
(d) Tongue licking Prompt the child to lick around their lips Before using honey, ensure that the child has no honey allergies and is over 12 months old The SLT may apply honey around the lips to elicit the child's movement or prompt the child to lick along a lollipop Encourage full circular motions around the lips Repeat the movement 10 times
(e) Tongue tip to cheek Prompt the child to press the tip of the tongue against the inside of the cheek Repeat on both sides Repeat the movement 10 times on each side

(c) *Tongue tip elevation*: Lifting the tongue tip up towards the alveolar ridge (the spot behind the top front teeth).
(d) *Tongue licking*: Licking around the lips or a lollipop to improve tongue mobility and coordination.
(e) *Tongue tip to cheek*: Pushing the tongue tip against the inside of the cheek, improving strength and lateral movement.

Examples of tongue exercises with step-by-step instructions to improve tongue mobility, strength, and coordination are presented in Table 5.5.

5.7.2 Factors Affecting Treatment Results

Several factors influence the effectiveness of behavioural and oral motor interventions:

(a) Cognitive and attention ability: Children with higher cognitive ability have better language understanding and better commitment to therapy. Children with appropriate attention spans demonstrate better responses to behavioural reinforcement and cueing techniques [4].
(b) Severity of neuromotor dysfunction: Children with mild or moderate neuromotor problems often receive greater benefit from behavioural and oral motor therapy than those with severe neuromotor problems because they may need additional medical intervention [15].
(c) Consistency and caregivers' participation: Practising regularly at home and having caregivers actively involved are key for children to learn and keep new skills [9, 56].
(d) Intensity and duration of therapy: Intensive and consistent therapy programs, such as daily or multi-week therapy sessions, will usually provide stronger and more persistent results [44, 52].
(e) Environmental generalisation: practicing new skills in different places, like at home, school, and clinics, will help children keep the therapy consistent [16].

5.8 Conclusion

For children with neurological or developmental disorders, evidence-based interventions, such as behavioural and oral motor therapy, are important to manage drooling. These approaches will improve both daily functioning and social well-being by targeting the motor and cognitive skills underlying saliva control. The integration of behavioural training, sensory activities, and structured oral exercises provides a strong foundation for non-invasive treatments, although ongoing support may be required to sustain therapeutic outcomes.

Appendix

HOMEWORK

DATE: ____________________ **NAME:** ____________________________

BREATHING

GOALS: ACTIVITIES:

JAW

GOALS: ACTIVITIES:

LIPS

GOALS: ACTIVITIES:

TONGUE

GOALS: ACTIVITIES:

HOMEWORK (Example)

DATE: ________________ **NAME:** __________________________

BREATHING

GOALS:
1. To improve nasal breathing.

ACTIVITIES:
1. Encourage the child to close his lips and hum his favourite song.
2. Use a finger to close the left nostril and breathe through the right nostril 10x; repeat the same for the right nostril.

JAW

GOALS:
1. To increase jaw strength and jaw stability.
2. To increase jaw grading.

ACTIVITIES:
1. Place a chewy tube on the left molars, ask the child to chew for 10x, and repeat the same on the right side.
2. Tug of war – Place a clean cloth near the molar, ask the child to bite and you can gently pull it.

LIPS

GOALS:
1. To increase lip strength.

ACTIVITIES:
1. Hold a tongue depressor or spatula on lips, make sure the child is not using teeth to bite on it; ask the child to hold it for 20x.

TONGUE

GOALS:
1. To increase tongue strength and tongue stability.

ACTIVITIES:
1. Move tongue to the left corner, then right corner of the mouth; repeat 10x.

References

1. Arslan SS, Demir N, Karaduman AA. Effect of a new treatment protocol called functional chewing training on chewing function in children with cerebral palsy: a double-blind randomised controlled trial. J Oral Rehabil. 2016;44(1):43–50. https://doi.org/10.1111/joor.12459.
2. Arvedson JC, Brodsky L, Lefton-Greif MA. Pediatric swallowing and feeding: assessment and management. 3rd ed. Plural Publishing; 2020.
3. Bavikatte G, Sit PL, Hassoon A. Management of drooling of saliva. Br J Med Pract. 2012;5(1):a507.
4. Brei TJ. Management of drooling. Semin Pediatr Neurol. 2003;10(4):265–70.
5. Chaléat-Valayer E, Porte M, Buchet-Poyau K, Roumenoff-Turcant F, D'Anjou M, Boulay C, Bernard J, Touzet S. Management of drooling in children with cerebral palsy: a French survey. Eur J Paediatr Neurol. 2016;20(4):524–31. https://doi.org/10.1016/j.ejpn.2016.04.010.
6. Clancy KJ, Hustad KC. Longitudinal changes in feeding among children with cerebral palsy between the ages of 4 and 7 years. Dev Neurorehabil. 2011;14(4):191–8. https://doi.org/10.3109/17518423.2011.568467.
7. Clawson EP, Kuchinski KS, Bach R. Use of behavioral interventions and parent education to address feeding difficulties in young children with spastic diplegic cerebral palsy. NeuroRehabilitation. 2007;22:397–406.
8. Crysdale WS, McCann C, Roske L, Joseph M, Semenuk D, Chait P. Saliva control issues in the neurologically challenged. Int J Pediatr Otorhinolaryngol. 2005;70(3):519–27. https://doi.org/10.1016/j.ijporl.2005.07.021.
9. Crysdale WS, McCann C, Roske L, Joseph M, Semenuk D, Chait P. Saliva control issues in the neurologically challenged: a 30-year experience in team management. Int J Pediatr Otorhinolaryngol. 2006;70(3):519–27.
10. Daniel SJ, Fayoux P, Bateman N, Boudewyns A, Brigger M, Chan CY, Chan K, Cheng A, Conley S, Kubba H, Lambert EM, Muntz H, Nuss R, Russell J, Rutter M, Schwarz Y, Spratley J, Thevasagayam R, Thompson D, et al. Comprehensive management of anterior drooling: an International Pediatric Otolaryngology Group (IPOG) consensus statement. Int J Pediatr Otorhinolaryngol. 2023;168:111500. https://doi.org/10.1016/j.ijporl.2023.111500.
11. De Bruijn TWP, Sohier J, Van Der Burg JJW. Outpatient treatment based on self-management strategies for chronic drooling in two children. J Dev Phys Disabil. 2017;29(5):735–55. https://doi.org/10.1007/s10882-017-9553-1.
12. De Weger WW, Bruinenberg VM, Van Der Lek EM, Gerrits JH, Van Lente L, Herpertz CE, Van Der Meulen GN, Sprikkelman AB, Koppelman GH, Kamps AW. Detection of salivary tryptase levels in children following oral food challenges. Int Arch Allergy Immunol. 2021;183(3):322–5. https://doi.org/10.1159/000519374.
13. Ekici B, Sigan S, Uzunhan T, Aydinli N, Eraslan E, Çaliskan M. Effects of oral motor therapy in children with cerebral palsy. Ann Indian Acad Neurol. 2013;16(3):342. https://doi.org/10.4103/0972-2327.116923.
14. Erasmus CE, Van Hulst K, Scheffer AR, Van Limbeek J, Van Den Hoogen FJ, Rotteveel JJ, Jongerius PH. What could predict effectiveness of botulinum toxin to treat drooling: a search for evidence of discriminatory factors on the level of body functions or structures. Eur J Paediatr Neurol. 2011;16(2):126–31. https://doi.org/10.1016/j.ejpn.2011.06.002.
15. Fairhurst CBR, Cockerill H. Management of drooling in children. Arch Dis Child Educ Pract Ed. 2011;96(1):25–30.
16. Fernandes AR, Dias BLS, Maia Filho HS. Sialorrhea in children with cerebral palsy. J Pediatr. 2016;92(6):549–58.
17. Garber J. Oral–motor function and feeding intervention. Phys Occup Ther Pediatr. 2013;33(1):111–38. https://doi.org/10.3109/01942638.2012.750864.
18. Greene Z, O'Donnell CP, Walshe M. Oral stimulation techniques in preterm infants—international research challenges. J Neonatal Nurs. 2013;19(4):168–74. https://doi.org/10.1016/j.jnn.2013.03.005.

19. Gupta A, Balasubramanian S, Bhavsar R. Efficacy of oral-sensory-motor intervention in the management for drooling of saliva in children with cerebral palsy–a cross-sectional study. Int J Health Sci Res. 2022;12(7):70–9. https://doi.org/10.52403/ijhsr.20220710.
20. Hall KD. Pediatric dysphagia resource guide. Singular; 2001.
21. Harding C, Faiman A, Wright J. Evaluation of an intensive desensitisation, oral tolerance therapy and hunger provocation program for children who have had prolonged periods of tube feeds. Int J Evid Based Healthc. 2010;8(4):268–76. https://doi.org/10.1111/j.1744-1609.2010.00184.x.
22. Holmberg KV, Hoffman MP, Karger S. Anatomy and physiology. Monogr Oral Sci. 2014;24:1–13. https://doi.org/10.1159/000358776.
23. Inal Ö, Arslan SS, Demir N, Yilmaz ÖT, Karaduman AA. Effect of functional chewing training on tongue thrust and drooling in children with cerebral palsy: a randomised controlled trial. J Oral Rehabil. 2017;44(11):843–9. https://doi.org/10.1111/joor.12544.
24. Kersner M, Wright JA. Speech and language therapy. London: Routledge; 2012.
25. Little SA, Kubba H, Hussain SS. An evidence-based approach to the child who drools saliva. Clin Otolaryngol. 2009;34(3):236–9. https://doi.org/10.1111/j.1749-4486.2009.01917.x. PMID: 19531173
26. Marinone S, Gaynor W, Johnston J, Mahadevan M. Castillo Morales Appliance Therapy in the treatment of drooling children. Int J Pediatr Otorhinolaryngol. 2017;103:129–32. https://doi.org/10.1016/j.ijporl.2017.10.020.
27. Meningaud J, Pitak-Arnnop P, Chikhani L, Bertrand J. Drooling of saliva: a review of the etiology and management options. Oral Surg Oral Med Oral Pathol Oral Radiol Endodontol. 2005;101(1):48–57. https://doi.org/10.1016/j.tripleo.2005.08.018.
28. Mikami M, et al. Evaluation of drooling parameters in children with oral motor dysfunction. Int J Pediatr Otorhinolaryngol. 2019;118:89–95.
29. Min K, Seo S, Woo H. Effect of oral motor facilitation technique on oral motor and feeding skills in children with cerebral palsy: a case study. BMC Pediatr. 2022;22(1):626. https://doi.org/10.1186/s12887-022-03674-8.
30. Mokhlesin M, Mirmohammadkhani M, Tohidast SA. The effect of Kinesio taping on drooling in children with intellectual disability: a double-blind randomised controlled study. Int J Pediatr Otorhinolaryngol. 2022;153:111017.
31. Montgomery J, McCusker S, Lang K, Grosse S, Mace A, Lumley R, Kubba H. Managing children with sialorrhoea (drooling): experience from the first 301 children in our saliva control clinic. Int J Pediatr Otorhinolaryngol. 2016;85:33–9. https://doi.org/10.1016/j.ijporl.2016.03.010.
32. Nayak M, Srinath SK, Azher U, Srinath S, More S, Goveas SR. Evaluation of efficacy of app-based oral motor therapy and behavior therapy in improving functions of oral musculature and oral hygiene in children with cerebral palsy: a randomized clinical trial. J Indian Soc Pedod Prev Dent. 2025;43(1):120–8. https://doi.org/10.4103/jisppd.jisppd_532_24.
33. Neurodevelopment and Disability, Dentistry, Plastic and Maxillofacial Surgery, & Speech Pathology. Saliva control in children. In: An information guide for families and clinicians; 1991. https://www.rch.org.au/uploadedfiles/main/content/plastic/salivabook.pdf.
34. Olsson SE, Chorney SR, Brown AT, Johnson RF, Kou Y. The role of speech therapy in sialorrhea management and quality of life: a retrospective study. Laryngosc Investig Otolaryngol. 2025;10(1):e70105. https://doi.org/10.1002/lio2.70105.
35. Ongkasuwan J, Chiou EH. Pediatric dysphagia: challenges and controversies. Springer International Publishing; 2018.
36. Orriëns LB, De Groot SAF, Van Der Burg JJW, Van Den Hoogen FJA, Van Hulst K, Erasmus CE. Interdisciplinary assessment and treatment of paediatric drooling: two decades of experience by the Nijmegen saliva control team reflected in a stepwise algorithm. Eur J Pediatr. 2024;183(9):3979–85. https://doi.org/10.1007/s00431-024-05658-5.
37. Orriëns LB, Van Aarle LGJM, Erasmus CE, Van Hulst K, Van Der Burg JJW. Social and emotional impact of anterior drooling in school-age children and young people with neurodevelopmental disabilities. Eur J Pediatr. 2024;183(10):4491–8. https://doi.org/10.1007/s00431-024-05714-0.

38. Palmer MM, Heyman MB, Zitzer C, Weinberg V, Glidden D, Dahlstrom C. The effects of sensory-based treatment of drooling in children. Phys Occup Ther Pediatr. 2009;18–18:85–95. https://doi.org/10.1080/J006v18n03_06.
39. Papandreou A, Mahony A, Breaks A, Absoud M, Fairhurst C. Comparative efficacy and side effect profiles of interventions for Pediatric saliva control: a cohort study. J Pediatr. 2023;265:113803. https://doi.org/10.1016/j.jpeds.2023.113803.
40. Pradon J, Barzic A, Lavadera ML, Khirani S, Canavesio C, Fleurence E, Labouret G, Aubertin G, Denamur S, Taytard J. Secretion management devices reduce hospitalizations for respiratory exacerbations in children with neurodisability. Respir Med. 2025;245:108183. https://doi.org/10.1016/j.rmed.2025.108183.
41. Reddihough DS, Johnson H. Assessment and management of saliva control problems in children and adults with neurological impairment. J Dev Phys Disabil. 1999;11(1):1–18.
42. Reddihough D, Johnson H, Ferguson E. The role of a saliva control clinic in the management of drooling. J Paediatr Child Health. 1992;28(5):395–7.
43. Redstone F, West JF. The importance of postural control for feeding. In: Lehman College, editor. The CE Posttest; 2004. p. 108–9.
44. Riva A, Amadori E, Vari MS, Spalice A, Belcastro V, Viri M, Capodiferro D, Romeo A, Verrotti A, Aiello MF, Bagnasco I, Battistella PA, Bergamoni S, Boldrini B, Bratta P, Brusaferro A, Brusco M, Burchiani B, Burdino E, et al. Impact and management of drooling in children with neurological disorders: an Italian Delphi consensus. Ital J Pediatr. 2022;48(1):118. https://doi.org/10.1186/s13052-022-01312-8.
45. Roque A, Perez-Jimenez M, Simões C, Carreira L, Silva FCE, Batalha N, Raimundo A, Lamy E. Effect of physical exercise on taste perception and saliva composition: an exploratory study. Food Res Int. 2025;221(Pt 3):117452. https://doi.org/10.1016/j.foodres.2025.117452.
46. Russo EF, Calabrò RS, Sale P, Vergura F, De Cola MC, Militi A, et al. Can muscle vibration be the future in the treatment of cerebral palsy-related drooling? Int J Med Sci. 2019;16(11):1447–52.
47. Santos MTBR, Manzano FS, Ferreira MCD, Masiero D. Development of a novel orofacial motor function assessment scale for children with cerebral palsy. J Dent Child. 2005;72(3):113–8.
48. Shapira J, Becker A, Moskovitz M. The management of drooling problems in children with neurological dysfunction: a review and case report. SCD Spec Care Dent. 1999;19(4):181–5.
49. Sjögreen L, Tulinius M, Kiliaridis S, Lohmander A. The effect of lip strengthening exercises in children and adolescents with myotonic dystrophy type 1. Int J Pediatr Otorhinolaryngol. 2010;74(10):1126–34. https://doi.org/10.1016/j.ijporl.2010.06.013.
50. Söyler AK, Arslan SS, Demir N, Karaduman AA, Düger T. Chewing and swallowing training in Coffin–Lowry syndrome: a case report. J Oral Rehabil. 2024;51(11):2500–2. https://doi.org/10.1111/joor.13820.
51. Thomas-Stonell N, Greenberg J. Three treatment approaches and clinical factors in the reduction of drooling. Dysphagia. 1988;3(2):73–8. https://doi.org/10.1007/BF02412423.
52. Van Der Burg JJW, Didden R, Engbers N, Jongerius PH, Rotteveel JJ. Self-management treatment of drooling: a case series. J Behav Ther Exp Psychiatry. 2009;40(1):106–19. https://doi.org/10.1016/j.jbtep.2008.05.001.
53. Van Hulst K, Van Den Engel-Hoek L, Geurts A, Jongerius P, Van Der Burg J, Feuth T, Van Den Hoogen F, Erasmus C. Development of the Drooling Infants and Preschoolers Scale (DRIPS) and reference charts for monitoring saliva control in children aged 0–4 years. Infant Behav Dev. 2018;50:247–56. https://doi.org/10.1016/j.infbeh.2018.01.004.
54. Vykuntaraju KN, Kalra V. Cerebral palsy and early stimulation. Jaypee Brothers Medical Publishers (P) Ltd.; 2014.
55. Willging JP, Miller CK, Cohen AP. Pediatric dysphagia: etiologies, diagnosis, and management. Plural Publishing; 2020.
56. Yam WKL, Yang HLC, Abdullah V, Chan CYL. Management of drooling for children with neurological problems in Hong Kong. Brain Dev. 2005;28(1):24–9. https://doi.org/10.1016/j.braindev.2005.03.008.

57. Yam WKL, Yang HLC, Abdullah V, Chan CYL. Management of drooling for children with neurological problems in Hong Kong. Brain Dev. 2006;28(1):24–9.
58. Yokochi K. Oral motor patterns during feeding in severely physically disabled children. Brain Dev. 1997;19(8):552–5.
59. Zamani SM, Naderifar E, Torabi MH, Kamali M. Non-medical treatments of drooling by speech and language pathologists in cerebral palsy children: a systematic review. J Iran Med Counc. 2024;7(4):599–613. https://doi.org/10.18502/jimc.v7i4.16622.

Pharmacological Management of Drooling in Children

6

Hannah Burns and Abigail Salcedo

6.1 Introduction

Drooling is considered a normal developmental phenomenon up to 18 months of age but becomes clinically significant when it persists beyond 4 years [1]. Problematic drooling is particularly common in children with cerebral palsy (CP) where reported prevalence ranges from 22 to 40% [2, 3]. Chronic sialorrhoea encompasses both anterior drooling and posterior loss of saliva into the pharynx. While anterior drooling is primarily associated with physical, social and psychological consequences that adversely affect quality of life, posterior drooling may contribute to aspiration, respiratory morbidity and impaired airway protection in vulnerable children. The etiology is multifactorial and most commonly reflects oral motor dysfunction—such as poor oromotor control, impaired lip closure, and postural abnormalities—rather than true hypersalivation [1, 4]. Management is therefore multidimensional and ideally undertaken by a multidisciplinary team, following a stepwise approach. Pharmacologic interventions are typically introduced when behavioral and conservative measures are insufficient and may serve as either a definitive treatment or a bridge to more invasive surgical options [5, 6]. A wide range of medications—including anticholinergic agents and botulinum injection

H. Burns (✉)
Faculty of Health, Medicine and Behavioural Sciences, University of Queensland, Brisbane, QLD, Australia

Department of Otorhinolaryngology Head and Neck Surgery, Queensland Children's Hospital, Children's Health Queensland, Brisbane, QLD, Australia
e-mail: Hannah.Burns@health.qld.gov.au

A. Salcedo
Department of Otolaryngology Head and Neck Surgery, Western Visayas Medical Center, Iloilo, Philippines
e-mail: assalcedo@alum.up.edu.ph

J. Saniasiaya (ed.), *An Overview of Drooling in Children*,
https://doi.org/10.1007/978-981-92-1850-9_6

Table 6.1 Stepwise approach to management of pediatric drooling

1. Rehabilitation and behavioral intervention
Speech and behavioral therapy
Posture and positioning
Oral appliances
2. Pharmacotherapy with anticholinergics
Glycopyrrolate
Scopolamine
Atropine
Trihexyphenidyl
3. Pharmacotherapy with botulinum injection
OnabotulinumtoxinA
AbobotulinumtoxinA
IncobotulinumtoxinA
RimabotulinumtoxinB
4. Surgery
Submandibular and/or parotid duct ligation
Submandibular duct relocation
Parotid duct relocation
Sublingual gland excision
Submandibular gland excision

therapies—are used in clinical practice, yet there remains no clear consensus regarding optimal drug selection, dosing, or duration of therapy [7]. This chapter reviews the pharmacologic management of pediatric drooling, with a focus on mechanisms of action, efficacy, safety profiles, and practical considerations to guide individualized treatment decisions. Table 6.1 describes a stepwise approach to the treatment of pediatric sialorrhea.

6.2 Anticholinergic Drugs

Anticholinergic agents are considered the first-line pharmacologic treatment for problematic drooling, particularly in pediatric populations. These drugs act by reversibly blocking cholinergic muscarinic receptors thereby reducing salivary flow, which is primarily driven by the parasympathetic autonomic nervous system [8]. Various anticholinergic medications studied and used for sialorrhea include glycopyrrolate, hyoscine hydrobromide, atropine, benztropine, and trihexyphenidyl (benzhexol hydrochloride). While effective in reducing saliva production, their antimuscarinic effects are not site-specific, often leading to a range of systemic side effects. These include behavioral changes—one of the most frequently reported adverse effects—as well as constipation, flushing, pupillary dilation or visual disturbances, and urinary retention [9]. Less commonly reported effects include xerostomia, sleep disturbances, and vomiting. These side effects have, in numerous cases, necessitated discontinuation of treatment, with several trials identifying adverse events as the most common reason for stopping therapy [10–12]. However, in one study, discontinuation was more often due to insufficient or diminished efficacy than to side effects [13]. Given the lack of consensus on optimal dosing and delivery methods, current recommendations emphasize initiating therapy at the lowest possible dose and titrating upward based on clinical response and tolerability [14].

Managing drooling continues to be a challenge. Although there are effective treatments to reduce saliva production, drooling may persist. Several factors can influence salivary flow rate, including medications, circadian rhythms, sensory stimulation, gender, age, psychological factors, and overall health.

Both botox injection and surgery are considered invasive. Anticholinergics offer a valuable noninvasive treatment and can be particularly beneficial in the following scenarios: (1) younger children who may still experience natural maturation of oral motor function—typically up to around 6 years of age—before more invasive treatments are considered; (2) older children with mild drooling issues; (3) children and families seeking to avoid surgery, preferring a nonoperative treatment option; and (4) children participating in behavioral programs, where reducing saliva volume can enhance the effectiveness and success of such interventions [15].

The following sections will examine each agent in detail, focusing on their efficacy in drooling reduction and associated rates of adverse effects.

6.2.1 Glycopyrrolate

Glycopyrrolate is the most extensively studied anticholinergic agent for managing sialorrhea and is often considered the first-line treatment, especially in children with neurological disorders. It is a quaternary ammonium compound with potent antisialogogue effects that selectively and prolongedly reduce salivary and sweat gland secretions by competitively inhibiting peripheral acetylcholine receptors. Unlike many other anticholinergics, glycopyrrolate poorly crosses the blood-brain barrier, minimizing central nervous system side effects [16]. It is available in oral and parenteral forms, with oral solutions preferred for drooling management due to precise dosing flexibility. An oral formulation was first approved by the US Food and Drug Administration (FDA) in 2010 for chronic severe drooling in children aged 3–16 years. In recent years, a case series of 18 patients under 3 years old with complex medical conditions have demonstrated that glycopyrrolate is an effective drug and can be used without major complications in this age group for a long period [17]. It has a rapid onset of action (15–30 min orally) and a duration of effect up to 8–12 h, making it particularly useful for nighttime symptoms [18, 19]. Its oral bioavailability is low (~10%) and variable, with food—especially high-fat meals—reducing absorption; thus, administration is recommended at least 1 h before or 2 h after meals [20].

Dosing Typical dosing starts at 0.02 mg/kg three times daily, titrated up in 0.02 mg/kg increments every 5–7 days based on efficacy and tolerability, with a maximum dose generally not exceeding 0.1 mg/kg three times daily or 1.5–3 mg per dose [21].

Glycopyrrolate is reported to be 5–6 times more potent than atropine for saliva reduction.

Efficacy Clinical studies have demonstrated improvements in drooling severity, caregiver burden, social interaction, and self-esteem in children treated long term with glycopyrrolate, though some patients may experience diminished effect or increased side effects over time eventually necessitating switching to an alternate treatment in most long-term users [13]. Multiple placebo-controlled trials have demonstrated glycopyrrolate's superiority in improving drooling outcomes [10, 22, 23]. A systematic review showed glycopyrrolate to have similar efficacy but higher tolerability than its comparators [24]. Comparison with scopolamine patch showed that both drugs cause significant reduction in the Drooling Impact Scale; however, scopolamine produced more problematic side effects leading to a greater chance of treatment cessation [11]. Parental engagement in treatment goals is essential to balance therapeutic benefits against side effects and optimize outcomes.

Precautions While effective at reducing drooling severity and frequency, glycopyrrolate is associated with dose-related adverse effects. Studies have demonstrated constipation as the predominant symptom [10, 11, 13, 23] and advised dosage adjustment and patient assessment, particularly within 4–5 days of initial administration or after a dose increase [25]. Another serious side effect noted is pseudo-obstruction, believed to result from decrease in intestinal motility that may have been caused or worsened by the medication [26]. Other common side effects include dry mouth, urinary retention, and visual disturbances. Behavioral changes and thickening of secretions have been noted, warranting caution in patients with compromised swallowing or posterior drooling [1, 26]. Glycopyrrolate should be used with caution in anyone with constipation, decreased intestinal motility and in those living in very warm to hot environments. Contraindications include conditions precluding anticholinergic use, such as glaucoma, intestinal obstruction, myasthenia gravis, and severe renal or hepatic impairment.

Duration of Treatment There is currently no consensus on how long should glycopyrrolate be used. On a prospective observational cohort, it was found out that participants' best response to glycopyrrolate was at a mean of 11.5 (SD 7.2) weeks [27]. Zanon [25] demonstrated that patients taking the drug for 24 months had more significant improvement in drooling compared to those who only took it for 12 months. Parents reported the greatest improvement in quality of life when the medication was used for 25–36 months [25].

Overall, glycopyrrolate's favorable efficacy and tolerability profile make it a cornerstone in the medical management of problematic drooling.

6.2.2 Scopolamine Hydrobromide

Scopolamine (hyoscine) is a tertiary amine antimuscarinic agent that exerts its effect by competitively antagonizing muscarinic acetylcholine receptors (M1–M5) throughout the parasympathetic nervous system. This drug reduces salivary secretion by blocking parasympathetic innervation to the salivary glands which makes it an effective antisialagogue. Because it is lipophilic and readily crosses the blood-brain barrier, scopolamine also has central nervous system (CNS) effects, a property that distinguishes it from quaternary antimuscarinics such as glycopyrrolate [24]. When administered orally or parenterally, its effects typically last 5–6 h. The transdermal formulation provides sustained systemic delivery over 48–72 h and is the most studied route in children [28, 29]. In a UK clinical practice survey, among the 98% of pediatricians who reported use of medication to manage sialorrhea, 85% used scopolamine patches as their first-line treatment, followed by glycopyrronium liquid as the second choice. This may be due to the convenience of a single transdermal patch lasting up to 3 days, compared to the need for 2–3 daily doses with oral alternatives [30].

Dosing The pediatric literature primarily reports on transdermal delivery. In clinical practice, a single patch is applied to hairless skin (commonly behind the ear) and replaced every 48–72 h. Because standard patches are manufactured for adults, pediatric providers often modify application by trimming patches or limiting the duration of wear to reduce systemic exposure in small children [28, 29]. Dosing in published reports is therefore heterogeneous, and no standardized weight-based regimen has been validated. A National Health System (NHS) guideline recommends age-based dosing of transdermal hyoscine hydrobromide patches, changed every 3 days (Table 6.2) [31]. To date, there is no established and universally accepted pediatric dosing schedule.

Efficacy Although available evidence is modest, scopolamine has shown consistent symptomatic benefit for pediatric drooling. Lewis and colleagues published a randomized, placebo-controlled, crossover study in 1994 in ten developmentally delayed children with excessive drooling using scopolamine transdermal patch [28]. Parents, caregivers, and therapists were asked to rate the amount of drooling using an observational scale. Over half of the enrolled patients reported at least a twofold

Table 6.2 Transdermal scopolamine pediatric dosing [31]

Hyoscine hydrobromide 1.5 mg patch
Patch placement: Behind ear
Age-based fractions:
1 month–3 years: ¼ patch
3–10 years: ½ patch
≥10 years: Full patch
Change interval: 48–72 h

reduction in drooling, and drooling was eliminated in one-third. Franco and colleagues used an oral formulation of scopolamine in a case series of four pediatric ICU patients.

Based on the Drooling Severity and Frequency Scale (DSFS), all four had improvement in frequency/severity of drooling at 24 h vs baseline [32]. Jongerius and colleagues in 2004 tried to compare scopolamine and botox in a controlled, open-label clinical trial. Drooling was evaluated at baseline, after 10 days of scopolamine application (changed every 72 h) and at different intervals up to 24 weeks after Botulinum Neurotoxin (BoNT) injections into the submandibular glands (SMG). Drooling was notably reduced by both interventions when compared to baseline levels. The effectiveness of scopolamine and BoNT fell within a comparable range, and no statistically significant differences in Drooling Quotient (DQ) were detected between the two treatments. Analysis of the Drooling Quotient (DQ) showed a 53% response rate to scopolamine [33]. Al Jeraisy and colleagues performed the largest pediatric study to date, involving 44 patients aged 3–14 years. They demonstrated significant reduction in severe/very severe drooling from 87.5% at baseline to 15.6% after ≥1 year of scopolamine therapy ($p < 0.001$) using DSFS. The study also showed significant reductions in emergency department visits (absolute risk reduction 27.6%) and hospital readmissions (35.7%) related to drooling management [29].

Precautions Scopolamine is contraindicated in patients with acute angle glaucoma and known sensitivity to scopolamine or other belladonna alkaloids or to any ingredient or component in the formulation or delivery system. Scopolamine demonstrates a significant side effect profile in pediatric populations. Up to 71.1% of patients experienced moderate to severe side effects when using scopolamine, leading to frequent discontinuation [28, 32]. Common adverse effects include xerostomia, pupillary dilatation and visual disturbances, behavioral changes, tachycardia, and urinary retention [24]. Some children had to discontinue their treatment with hyoscine patches due to skin reactions to the patch adhesive [11, 34]. Side effects were observed as early as within 3 days of application [33]. A comparative study between scopolamine patches and glycopyrrolate showed that scopolamine caused more side effects, leading nearly half of the parents (45%) to stop treatment, compared to only 15% in the glycopyrrolate group [11].

Conclusion In clinical practice, scopolamine is a commonly used and effective option for managing sialorrhea in pediatric patients, particularly due to the convenience of its transdermal patch formulation and its ability to significantly reduce drooling severity and associated healthcare needs. However, its use is tempered by a lack of standardized pediatric dosing and a relatively high rate of adverse effects, which often necessitate treatment discontinuation. As such, while scopolamine remains a valuable therapeutic tool, careful patient selection, close monitoring, and consideration of alternative agents like glycopyrrolate are essential to optimizing both safety and efficacy.

6.2.3 Atropine

Atropine is another nonselective muscarinic antagonist that blocks saliva production by targeting M3 muscarinic receptors in the salivary glands, making it effective for the management of drooling in pediatric patients [35]. Like other nonselective anticholinergics, atropine acts systemically, or topically via sublingual route, and can inhibit other cholinergic functions (e.g., in the gut, bladder, eyes), which underlies much of its side-effect profile. Compared to glycopyrrolate, hyoscine, trihexyphenidyl, and benztropine, the appearance of atropine in the drooling literature is far more recent [9].

There is currently no approved oral formulation, but the off-label use of sublingual atropine (SLA) ophthalmic drops is favored because it allows more localized effect and less systemic absorption compared with oral or parenteral administration. Indeed, a meta-analysis suggested that sublingual delivery offers greater reductions in salivary flow versus oral or subcutaneous routes [36]. The onset of action was found to be 15 to 30 min, and the duration of action was approximately 4 h [37]. An early phase 1 study on a mucoadhesive topical oral gel formulation has demonstrated safe and satisfactory pharmacologic profile giving promising results [38].

Dosing As a relatively new agent in this context, the recommended dosing and role of atropine in treatment are still being established. Because evidence is limited and largely observational, dosing regimens vary across studies. In the largest ($N = 178$) and most recent retrospective review of patients (age < 22 yo) who were given atropine, the most common starting dose was atropine 1% drops, two total drops per day, regardless of age or weight at the start of therapy and ranged up to 12 drops per day. No significant difference between average starting and final mg/day when adjusted for patient weight [39].

Efficacy The evidence base for the efficacy of atropine in pediatric drooling is modest and largely observational but suggests benefit in many cases. There are two prospective studies and one retroprospective study in children to date. Dias et al. [35] conducted an open-label clinical trial involving children with cerebral palsy. Twenty-five out of 33 completed the study, and there was significant decrease in the Drooling Impact Scale from 61.8 to 25.6 ($p < 0.001$) after 30 days of treatment. Overall, 92.3% had improvement in drooling [35]. In another study, Norderyd et al. used a prospective single-system design in which 19 children served as their own controls, with 11 completing the trial. There was significant improvement in the Visual Analogue Scale (VAS) ratings from baseline to once-daily treatment (74 vs 48, $p = 0.05$), and from once-daily to twice-daily dosing (48 vs 32, $p = 0.026$), showing regardless of whether atropine was administered one or two times per day, a positive effect was reflected in the parents' assessment of their child's drooling. A total of 81.8% of patients showed decreased salivary secretion rates [40]. Lastly, in a retrospective chart review, Azapagasi et al. [41] evaluated 25 hospitalized children treated with SLA for 7 days, with outcome data available for 20 patients. A significant improvement in 95% of the participants was observed as early as day 2 of using atropine based on the Teacher Drooling Scale, a 5-point rating system [41].

Precautions Studies suggest that SLA has a low incidence of side effects, likely due to its localized action on the salivary glands and minimal systemic absorption [37]. No serious adverse effects have been identified in the small body of literature available for SLA [35, 40, 41]. Given its anticholinergic action, atropine can produce a range of side effects such as mild dry mouth [35, 39], irritability [39] constipation, flushing, pupillary dilation or visual disturbances, and urinary retention [9]. Potential serious adverse effects from atropine which may include ataxia, delirium, coma, and respiratory failure [42] have not been reported in the reviewed literature. Notably, in two studies, parents reported an initial reduction in drooling during the course of treatment, followed by an increase toward the end of the study period [40] and approximately 1 week after discontinuation of the medication [41]. Most studies conducted had short duration, limited monitoring, or small sample size, and this may have affected the rate of side effects reported.

A specific challenge with SLA relates to the off-label use of atropine eye drops delivered sublingually, where inaccurate dosing is a significant concern. Variability in drop size, administration technique, and absorption can lead to unintended overdosing or underdosing, particularly in young children. Given these uncertainties, careful consideration and heightened clinical caution are advised when using SLA in pediatric populations, with close attention to dosing accuracy, caregiver education, and monitoring for potential systemic effects.

Conclusion SLA is cheap, accessible, easy to deliver, noninvasive and has fast onset. These and the reduced systemic absorption, minimal reported adverse effects to date, and the rapid onset of drying following sublingual administration of atropine make it a promising option for the treatment of sialorrhea in children. However, evidence supporting this off-label use remains limited, with studies generally involving small patient cohorts. Its use is further constrained by non-standardised dosing regimens, short mucosal contact time, the potential for medication errors, and the risk of systemic adverse effects [38]. While current findings suggest a promising role for SLA in the treatment of sialorrhea in children and young adults with neurodevelopmental disorders, further high-quality research is clearly needed.

6.2.4 Trihexyphenidyl/Benzhexol

Another anticholinergic used as an off-label treatment for drooling is trihexyphenidyl (also marketed as benzhexol hydrochloride) which has traditionally been deployed for movement disorders and widely used for adults with dystonia. Although no RCTs have been conducted to date, a few observational studies and case series provide insight into its efficacy and tolerability [27, 43, 44].

Mechanism of Action Trihexyphenidyl exerts its effects by competitive antagonism of central and peripheral muscarinic acetylcholine receptors, thereby reducing parasympathetic stimulation. Its anticholinergic action decreases salivary secretion from the salivary glands, accounting for its peripheral effect on drooling. Additionally, there is evidence that trihexyphenidyl may improve drooling through a central mechanism—enhancing motor control and coordination of oropharyngeal muscles involved in swallowing. Improved expressive language and oral motor function observed in some children may reflect this central action, distinguishing it from purely peripheral antisialagogues such as glycopyrrolate [44].

Dosing Dosing data in children are limited and largely off label for drooling. In the study by [43], comparable clinical efficacy was observed with 2 mg twice daily and 2 mg three times daily regardless of patient's weight. Carranza-del Rio et al. [44] started at a mean initial dose of 0.095 mg/kg/day in children (range 1–18 years) and titrated upward by 10–20% every 2 weeks, with a mean maximum dose reached of approximately 0.55 mg/kg/day. NHS guidelines mention under-10 years to start 1 mg twice daily and increase to 2 mg twice daily as tolerated and those over 10 years to go as high as 3 mg twice daily [31]. As with most anticholinergic therapies, dosing must be customized, titrated slowly considering tolerability, and individualized based on response and adverse effects.

Efficacy Evidence for trihexyphenidyl in drooling management is largely derived from observational data. An early prospective study done in 1990 showed 85% of the patients had improved drooling median rates posttreatment with trihexyphenidyl [43]. In a retrospective study done in 2011 on 101 children with CP, 60.4% reported benefit in sialorrhea reduction. However, applying these findings in clinical practice may be difficult since the study involved patients treated for both sialorrhea and dystonia [44]. Finally, a prospective observational study in 2020 tried to compare the efficacy of trihexyphenidyl, glycopyrrolate, and scopolamine. Overall response rates at the time of best response were 75%, 85%, and 65%, respectively. With trihexyphenidyl, best drooling response was recorded at a mean of 5 weeks after commencement of treatment. Glycopyrrolate performed best overall as it had the lowest failure rate and fewest side effects. Factors such as lower baseline drooling scores, non-oral feeding, limited or absent speech, and poor head control were associated with a poorer response to therapy [27]. Overall, while many clinicians report anecdotal benefit, trihexyphenidyl's magnitude of effect on drooling specifically is variable, and there is no large-scale randomized controlled trial strictly for drooling.

Precautions As with all antimuscarinic agents, documented side effects include constipation, dry mouth, urinary retention, and behavioral changes as the most common [27, 44]. Eighty-eight percent of carers reported at least one adverse side effect presumed due to trihexyphenidyl based on one study [27]. In another study, 44% of patients developed their first side effect at doses lower than 0.4 mg/kg/day, and

Table 6.3 Comparison of anticholinergic medications for pediatric drooling [21, 31, 39]

Medication	Route(s)	Typical dosing (pediatric)	Key advantages	Common adverse effects
Glycopyrrolate	Oral	Start 0.02 mg/kg TID titrated in 0.02 mg/kg increments every 5–7 days; max 0.1 mg/kg TID or 1.5–3 mg/dose	Best studied; does not cross blood-brain barrier; FDA-approved	Constipation, dry mouth, urinary retention, visual disturbances, thickening of saliva, behavioral changes
Scopolamine (hyoscine hydrobromide)	Transdermal (1.5 mg system)	Age-based patch fractions every 48–72 h (see Table 6.2)	Convenient patch; long duration	Xerostomia, pupillary dilatation and visual disturbances, behavioral changes, tachycardia, urinary retention [24]
Atropine	Sublingual (off label)	1% drops; typically 2–12 drops/day	Rapid onset; minimal systemic exposure and minimal reported adverse effects	Dry mouth, irritability
Trihexyphenidyl	Oral	< 10 years old—start 1 mg BID, increase to 2 mg BID as tolerated > 10 years old—as high as 3 mg BID	Central + peripheral benefit	Behavioral change, constipation, urinary retention, dry mouth

BID twice a day, *TID* thrice a day

treatment discontinuation was as high as 8% due to intolerable side effects [44]. One case report described an 8-year-old child with CP and long-term hypomotility issues on trihexyphenidyl for drooling who developed acute colonic pseudo-obstruction and needed to undergo emergency laparotomy and ileostomy, emphasizing the need to consider gastrointestinal motility risk [45].

Conclusion Trihexyphenidyl appears to offer a clinically meaningful reduction in drooling for many patients, though the supporting evidence is limited to observational studies and case series. Its dual mechanism—reducing salivary secretion through peripheral antimuscarinic activity and enhancing oral motor control via central effects—may explain its broader benefit compared with purely peripheral agents. However, the lack of randomized controlled trials and methodological limitations, such as heterogeneous study populations including patients treated for both dystonia and sialorrhea, constrain the strength of current evidence. Adverse effects are common like other anticholinergic drugs. While trihexyphenidyl can be an effective and accessible option for managing drooling, its use should be individualized, closely monitored for tolerability, and reserved for cases where the anticipated benefits outweigh the potential risks. A summary of anticholinergic medications in children for management of drooling is seen in Table 6.3.

6.3 Botulinum Toxin

Introduction The anaerobic bacterium *Clostridium botulinum* produces seven antigenically distinct neurotoxins, types A through G. All are potent neuroparalytic agents and similar in structure, but type A (BoNT-A) is thought to have greater anticholinergic effect at the neuromuscular junction. It has emerged over the past two decades as an effective, minimally invasive intervention to reduce drooling by temporarily reducing salivary gland output. Initially used in adults with neurological conditions such as Parkinson's disease and amyotrophic lateral sclerosis [46, 47], its success led to pediatric applications in the early 2000s [48, 49], and it is now supported by extensive clinical experience, randomized controlled trials, and systematic reviews as a standard of care for pediatric sialorrhea [50–54].

6.3.1 Mechanism of Action

BoNT-A exerts its effect by inhibiting the release of acetylcholine from presynaptic cholinergic nerve terminals at the neuroglandular junction. It cleaves the SNAP-25 protein of the SNARE complex, thereby preventing vesicular fusion and neurotransmitter release [55, 56]. This blockade leads to functional denervation of the salivary gland's parasympathetic input and consequently decreases glandular secretion. The effect is reversible as new synaptic terminals regenerate over a period of approximately 3–6 months [57]. Histological studies confirm glandular atrophy, reduced acinar density, and diminished secretory granules following injection, consistent with reduced salivary flow [55]. Function is restored gradually as cholinergic activity resumes, which underlies the temporary but repeatable clinical benefit observed with serial treatments.

Table 6.4 Botulinum toxin formulations and dosing used in pediatric sialorrhea [58, 60, 16, 53]

Toxin type	Brand name	Typical dose per SMG (U)	Typical dose per parotid gland (U)	Typical total dose range
OnabotulinumtoxinA	BOTOX®	10–50 [60]	10–50 [60]	50–100 [60]
AbobotulinumtoxinA	Dysport®	15–75 [60]	15–75 [60]	100–140 [60]
IncobotulinumtoxinA	Xeomin®	4–15 (weight-based) [77]	6–22.5 (weight-based) [77]	20–75 (weight-based) [77]
RimabotulinumtoxinB	Myobloc®	250–1000 [60]	400–1000 [60]	

U unit

6.3.2 Dosing and Injection Protocols

Dosing strategies for BoNT-A in pediatric sialorrhea have varied across studies, reflecting differences in toxin formulation, injection technique, and patient age. The two most marketed types of BoNT-A are onabotulinumtoxinA (BOTOX®) and abobotulinumtoxinA (Dysport®). The majority of available literature is on BOTOX®. Early investigations by Suskind and Tilton [49] and Jongerius et al. [48, 59] established efficacy using total doses ranging from 30 to 70 units of onabotulinumtoxinA divided between the parotid and SMG. Alrefai [58] meanwhile demonstrated that 100 to 140 units of abobotulinumtoxin A were safe and effective in the pediatric population. An international consensus statement guideline from 2010 recommends 10–50 U per gland (BOTOX®) and 15–75 U (Dysport®) [60]. Berweck et al. [52] showed a conservative body weight-dependent dosing approach using a total of 20–75 U, divided among four glands, of incobotulinumtoxinA (Xeomin®) for repeated treatment is safe while attaining good efficacy.

Subsequent controlled studies refined dosing to weight-based regimens of approximately 1–2 units/kg per gland [57, 61], while some followed a standard of 25 U per gland either SMG only or including parotid with doses not exceeding a total of 100 U [50, 62]. A systematic review revealed that in two-gland studies, most participants received 50 U of BoNT-A, while in four-gland studies, doses of 60–100 U were most common [53]. The effect appears to be dose-dependent, as one study reported the need for reinjection just 1 month after an initial total dose of 15.5 U [63], while doses exceeding 100 U have been associated with adverse effects such as dysphagia [64]. Furthermore, a randomized placebo-controlled trial with a small population showed that low dose BoNT-A (<50 U total) showed decrease in salivary flow rate but no improvement in subjective scales from carers [61]. Recommendations for dosing and injection sites are outlined in Table 6.4.

Careful dilution and injection technique are essential when administering botulinum toxin to maximize efficacy and minimize extraglandular spread. A common approach involves diluting 100 units in 1–2 mL of saline, with injection volumes of 0.25–0.5 mL per gland to reduce the risk of diffusion beyond the target area. Some authors recommend using larger volumes—up to 1–1.5 mL per gland—to promote broader distribution within the glandular parenchyma, though this may increase the risk of unintended effects such as dysphagia [65]. The onset of effect generally occurs within 5–7 days, with maximal benefit at 2–4 weeks and a duration of action of 3–6 months [56, 60]. Repeat injections can be performed safely at intervals of approximately 4 to 6 months for ongoing symptom control [53, 62].

6.3.3 Efficacy

BoNT-A has demonstrated robust efficacy in the management of pediatric sialorrhea across a wide range of objective and subjective outcome measures. Early prospective and controlled studies showed significant reductions in salivary flow rates and caregiver-rated drooling severity following BoNT-A injections [48, 49, 59, 66], findings that were subsequently confirmed by randomized, double-blind, placebo-controlled trials reporting improvements in drooling frequency, bib use, and health-related quality of life [52, 58, 61, 62]. These benefits were reinforced by systematic reviews focusing on pediatric populations, including those by Rodwell et al. [67] and Heikel et al. [53], showing positive treatment effects across multiple validated measures. Randomized studies report peak efficacy of botulinum toxin within 4–8 weeks postinjection [48, 68], with effects typically lasting 19–33 weeks (median ~ 22 weeks) [69] and some children experiencing benefits for up to a year [62]. Minimal waning of effect within the first 4 months supports the feasibility of maintaining control of sialorrhea with up to three treatments annually [52].

Beyond physical symptom reduction, BoNT-A has been associated with meaningful psychosocial benefits; improvements in social interaction and parental perceptions of physical appearance, family relationships, and overall life satisfaction have been reported in children with CP [70, 71], although changes in measured self-esteem have been less consistently demonstrated [70].

Repeated botulinum toxin injections can maintain efficacy, though the greatest therapeutic benefit is often seen after the first dose. Reported success rates decline over time—74.0% after the first injection, compared to 41.6% and 45.8% after the second and third, respectively [72]. This waning effect may reflect adaptive changes in glandular function, altered neuromuscular sensitivity, or patient habituation, though definitive mechanisms remain unclear. One proposed explanation is the development of neutralizing antibodies (nAbs) against the toxin, which may reduce its clinical effectiveness over time [73]. In such cases, switching to a different botulinum toxin formulation (e.g., from onabotulinumtoxinA to abobotulinumtoxinA or incobotulinumtoxinA) has been suggested as a potential strategy to overcome resistance and restore therapeutic response [74, 75].

6.3.4 Safety and Precautions

BoNT-A injections are generally safe and well tolerated in pediatric populations. Reported adverse effects are usually mild and transient. One or more adverse events following injection is common in studies [53], and there was one terminated randomized controlled trial due to serious adverse events [76]. Mild adverse effects like local pain, soreness, injection-site swelling, thickened saliva, or dry mouth have previously been reported in 10%–45% of the treatment series with BoNT-A and in 30%–40% with BoNT-B [68]. Other uncommon yet possible effects are transient flu-like symptoms [59] or respiratory infections [49, 52].

Most major risks associated with BoNT-A are locoregional effects secondary to unintended diffusion to nearby muscles. Research on BTX-A diffusion has shown that it can spread beyond the fascial planes [78]. Because of this diffusion, dysphagia can occur, especially at higher doses or following four-gland injections, but is typically self-limited [58, 59, 63, 69, 79]. Precautions should be observed in children with significant baseline dysphagia or compromised airway protection, as they may be at higher risk for aspiration. Pre-procedure evaluation by a multidisciplinary team—including speech and language therapy, otolaryngology, and neurology—is strongly recommended. Posttreatment monitoring for hydration, nutrition, and swallowing safety is also essential.

One notable effect is the thickening of salivary secretions, which occurs as BoNT blocks parasympathetic input to the salivary glands. This reduces the production of watery, serous saliva and may shift the balance toward sympathetically mediated secretion, which is more viscous and mucous-rich. In patients with impaired swallowing or limited mobility, this can lead to oropharyngeal pooling, mucus plugging, and potentially increased aspiration risk [80]. A study by Khan in 2011 documented a case of aspiration pneumonia prompting prolonged hospitalization which did not affect caregiver satisfaction and desire to repeat the procedure. Related to thickened saliva, abscess formation, although very rare, has been reported following glandular injection. This may result not only from injection-related inflammation or breach of aseptic technique but also from salivary stasis within the gland, which creates a favorable environment for bacterial overgrowth and infection [80].

Saliva's protective roles include buffering acids, antimicrobial action, and self-cleaning of teeth. Reduction of saliva production can increase the risk of dental caries and other oral health issues if dental hygiene is neglected. Patient receiving botulinum injection for drooling should be advised to maintain excellent oral hygiene and have regular dental follow-ups to prevent these potential problems [81].

Serious complications are exceedingly rare. One study had to be terminated early because one participant developed marked dysphagia with poor oral intake and rapid weight loss, while another experienced significant worsening of speech for several weeks without improvement in drooling [76].

Clinicians should also be aware of any BoNT-A injections given at other sites within the previous 4–6 months and coordinate care with other treating providers. Iatrogenic botulism is a rare but serious complication of excessive botulinum toxin exposure thought to result from systemic absorption of the neurotoxin, leading to generalized neuromuscular weakness and possible systemic myopathy with bulbar and respiratory involvement in severe cases. Inadvertent overdose, high cumulative dosing, short injection intervals, and dosing errors, particularly in pediatric and neurologic populations, are possible causes. Although not reported with sialorrhea treatment alone, this risk is an important consideration in children with CP who may

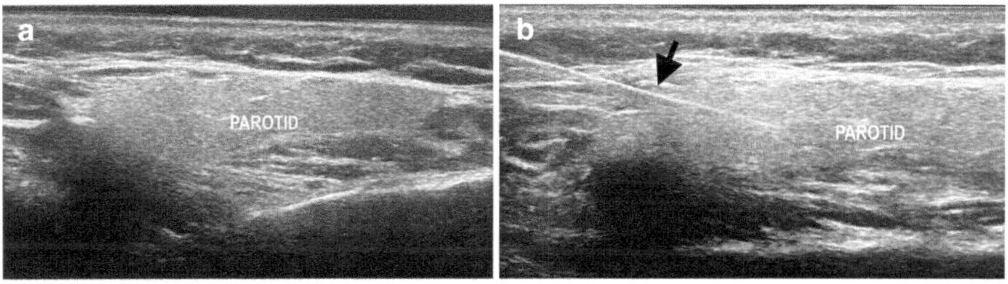

Fig. 6.1 (**a**). Sonography of the parotid gland, (**b**). Arrow showing needle in parotid parenchyma

receive botulinum toxin for multiple indications, such as spasticity and drooling, resulting in increased cumulative exposure. New or worsening dysphagia, generalized weakness, or fatigue following injections should raise concern for possible systemic toxin effects rather than isolated local diffusion. Management involves prompt supportive care and, in moderate to severe cases, administration of botulinum antitoxin with close monitoring for respiratory compromise [82, 83].

6.3.5 Ultrasound Guidance on BoNT Injection

Inaccurate administration of BoNT to the salivary glands risks damaging adjacent structures, including the facial nerve and carotid artery, while inadvertent injection into the masseter and pharyngeal muscles can result in weakness in chewing and dysphagia. Consequently, ultrasound guidance has become the standard approach for pediatric BoNT-A injections. By providing real-time visualization of gland anatomy, vascular structures, and needle placement, ultrasonography ensures precise intraglandular delivery and minimizes injury to surrounding tissues. Evidence suggests this modality improves procedural accuracy and efficacy, maintaining an exceptionally low overall complication rate of 0.6% when performed by pediatric otolaryngologists [79, 84].

The superiority of this technique was quantified in a cadaveric study comparing ultrasound-guided versus landmark-based injections. Accuracy for the parotid gland was 95.83% with ultrasound compared to 79.17% using landmarks; for the SMG, accuracy was 91.67% versus 50.00%, respectively [85]. While the difference for the parotid gland was not statistically significant, the results confirm that blind injection is unreliable for the SMG due to anatomical variability. Accordingly, international consensus statements advocate for ultrasound-guided injection as the best practice for pediatric sialorrhea management [60] (Fig. 6.1).

6.3.6 Two-Gland Versus Four-Gland Injection Strategies

There is currently no consensus on the optimal number of glands to inject for sialorrhea management, though the physiological roles of the glands often guide the strategy. The

SMG are responsible for approximately 70% of resting saliva production, while the parotid glands mainly contribute to stimulated saliva [86]. Early studies focused on bilateral SMG to target resting drooling while preserving parotid function for bolus lubrication during meals [48, 59, 69, 70]. However, later works have shown that combining parotid and submandibular injections (four-gland technique) provided superior and longer-lasting drooling control, particularly in severe cases [52, 57, 61, 62].

Some authors reserve four-gland injections for patients with severely inadequate swallowing mechanisms, suspected aspiration, or those refractory to submandibular treatment alone. Scheffer [69] cautions against combined injections in children who are fed orally, as diminished lubrication could impair feeding in patients where ample saliva is just barely enough. Lin et al. [87] proposed a compromise, injecting one parotid and the contralateral SMG to preserve at least 50% of saliva production, theoretically minimizing side effects..

Studies directly comparing two- and four-gland techniques are quite limited. To date, we found three randomized controlled studies, two of which support the safety and superior efficacy of four-gland injections [49, 68, 76], albeit with small sample sizes. Suskind and Tilton [49] demonstrated a significant difference in outcomes, reporting only a 30% response rate when injecting the SMG alone compared to an 80% response rate with the four-gland approach. Møller's [68] study evaluated escalating doses of botulinum toxin injected into two glands vs four glands and found that the highest combined-dose regimen (30 U per SMG and 30 U per parotid) produced the greatest improvement in drooling scores and the largest reduction in salivary flow rate.

Despite these findings, a definitive superiority remains difficult to prove statistically due to methodological heterogeneity. A 2024 scoping review by Orriens, which examined 7 articles on two-gland and 21 articles on four-gland injections, concluded that while substantial evidence exists for both techniques, the lack of standardization in patient populations and outcome measures makes it impossible to directly compare their effectiveness. However, the prevailing research suggests that four-gland injections are likely superior in efficacy, albeit with a slightly increased risk of transient swallowing difficulties. Therefore, the choice between techniques requires balancing the severity of drooling against the patient's feeding status: four-gland injections yield greater reduction in flow, but individualized dosing is critical to maintain the safety-efficacy balance.

6.3.7 Combined BoNT Injection and Surgical Treatment

There is emerging evidence supporting the combined use of botulinum toxin injections with surgical interventions such as submandibular duct ligation or sublingual gland excision for the treatment of sialorrhea. This multimodal approach can enhance efficacy in children with severe drooling who may not fully respond to a single modality. Calim et al. [89] describe a protocol involving staggered botulinum toxin A injections into the parotid and submandibular glands prior to four-duct ligation as part of a comprehensive treatment strategy. Similarly, Calim et al. [88]

reported combining intraparotid BoNT-A injection with submandibular duct rerouting and sublingual gland excision, demonstrating improved outcomes in refractory cases. These findings suggest that for select patients, combination therapy may offer superior symptom control compared to monotherapy.

6.4 Conclusion

BoNT-A injection has become a well-established and effective treatment for pediatric sialorrhea, supported by more than two decades of clinical experience, randomized controlled trials, and systematic reviews. The therapy is safe, reversible, and effective, offering substantial improvements in drooling control, social participation, and respiratory health for children with cerebral palsy and related disorders. Optimal outcomes are achieved through ultrasound-guided administration, individualized dosing, and interdisciplinary aftercare. It is well-tolerated with most adverse effects being mild, transient, and related to local diffusion. Overall, it represents a cornerstone therapy for moderate to severe pediatric sialorrhea, particularly when conservative and anticholinergic therapy are insufficient, though continued efforts toward standardization of protocols and outcome measures are needed to further refine best practice.

References

1. Blasco PA, Allaire JH. Drooling in the developmentally disabled: management practices and recommendations. Consortium on drooling. Dev Med Child Neurol. 1992;34(10):849–62.
2. Parkes J, Hill N, Platt MJ, Donnelly C. Oromotor dysfunction and communication impairments in children with cerebral palsy: a register study. Dev Med Child Neurol. 2010;52(12):1113–9. https://doi.org/10.1111/j.1469-8749.2010.03772.x.
3. Reid SM, McCutcheon J, Reddihough DS, Johnson HM. Prevalence and predictors of drooling in 7- to 14-year-old children with cerebral palsy: a population study. Dev Med Child Neurol. 2012;54(11):1032–6. https://doi.org/10.1111/j.1469-8749.2012.04382.x.
4. Erasmus CE, Van Hulst K, Rotteveel LJ, Jongerius PH, Van Den Hoogen FJ, Roeleveld N, Rotteveel JJ. Drooling in cerebral palsy: hypersalivation or dysfunctional oral motor control? Dev Med Child Neurol. 2009;51(6):454–9. https://doi.org/10.1111/j.1469-8749.2008.03243.x.
5. Little SA, Kubba H, Hussain SSM. An evidence-based approach to the child who drools saliva. Clin Otolaryngol. 2009;34(3):236–9. https://doi.org/10.1111/j.1749-4486.2009.01917.x.
6. Glader L, Delsing C, Hughes A, Parr J, Pennington L, Reddihough D, Van Hulst K, Van Der Burg J. AACPDM care pathway for sialorrhea in cerebral palsy. Am Acad Cereb Palsy Dev Med. 2017. Available at: http://www.aacpdm.org/publications/care-pathways/sialorrhea. Accessed 6 Aug 2025.
7. Varley LP, Denieffe S, O'Gorman C, Murphy A, Gooney M. A systematic review of non-invasive and invasive sialorrhoea management. J Clin Nurs. 2019;28(23–24):4190–206. https://doi.org/10.1111/jocn.15009.
8. Tscheng DZ. Sialorrhea—therapeutic drug options. Ann Pharmacother. 2002;36(11):1785–90. https://doi.org/10.1345/aph.1C019.
9. You P, Strychowsky J, Gandhi K, Chen BA. Anticholinergic treatment for sialorrhea in children: a systematic review. Paediatr Child Health. 2022;27(2):82–7. https://doi.org/10.1093/pch/pxab051.

10. Fayoux P, Dinomais M, Shaw H, Villain F, Schwartz D, Rondeau S, Letellier G, Auvin S. Glycopyrronium 320 μg/mL in children and adolescents with severe sialorrhoea and neurodisabilities: a randomized, double-blind, placebo-controlled trial. Dev Med Child Neurol. 2024;66(7):910–8. https://doi.org/10.1111/dmcn.15841.
11. Parr JR, Todhunter E, Pennington L, Stocken D, Cadwgan J, O'Hare AE, Tuffrey C, Williams J, Cole M, Colver AF. Drooling reduction intervention randomised trial (DRI): comparing the efficacy and acceptability of hyoscine patches and glycopyrronium liquid on drooling in children with neurodisability. Arch Dis Child. 2018;103(4):371–6. https://doi.org/10.1136/archdischild-2017-313763.
12. Zeller RS, Lee HM, Cavanaugh PF Jr, Davidson J. Safety and efficacy of glycopyrrolate oral solution for management of pathologic drooling in pediatric patients with cerebral palsy and other neurologic conditions. Ther Clin Risk Manag. 2012;8:25–32. https://doi.org/10.2147/TCRM.S27362.
13. Orriëns LB, Verhoeven WMA, Rijkers GT, Keunen JEE, van Hulst K, Rotteveel JJ, van der Burg J, Roodbol PF, van Limbeek J, Jongerius PH. The when, why, and how of using glycopyrronium to diminish drooling in children with neurodevelopmental disabilities: implications for clinical practice. Eur J Paediatr Neurol. 2024;51:24–31. https://doi.org/10.1016/j.ejpn.2024.05.004.
14. McGeachan AJ, McDermott CJ. Management of oral secretions in neurological disease. Pract Neurol. 2017;17(2):96–103. https://doi.org/10.1136/practneurol-2016-001515.
15. Reddihough D, Reid SM, Plover C. Evaluation of glycopyrrolate in the treatment of chronic drooling. Degener Neurol Neuromuscul Dis. 2011;1:3–7. https://doi.org/10.2147/DNND.S16084.
16. US Food and Drug Administration Cuvposa® (glycopyrrolate oral solution): US prescribing information. US Food and Drug Administration. 2010. Available at: https://www.accessdata.fda.gov/drugsatfda_docs/label/2010/022571s000lbl.pdf. Accessed 15 Oct 2025.
17. Lovardi E, De Ioris MA, Lettori D, Geremia C, Staccioli S, Della Bella G, Scrocca R, Scarselli A, Aversa M, De Peppo F, Campana A, Castelli E. Glycopyrrolate for drooling in children with medical complexity under three years of age. Ital J Pediatr. 2022;48(1):2. https://doi.org/10.1186/s13052-021-01195-1.
18. Hodding JH, Kraus DM, Taketomo CK. Pediatric dosage handbook. Hudson: Lexi-Comp; 2009.
19. Cada DJ, Levien TL, Baker DE. Formulary drug reviews—glycopyrrolate oral solution. Hosp Pharm. 2010;45(11):939–43.
20. Rautakorpi P, Manner T, Ali-Melkkilä T, Kaila T, Olkkola KT, Kanto J. Pharmacokinetics and oral bioavailability of glycopyrrolate in children. Pharmacol Toxicol. 1998;83(3):132–4. https://doi.org/10.1111/j.1600-0773.1998.tb01456.x.
21. Garnock-Jones KP. Glycopyrrolate oral solution: for chronic, severe drooling in pediatric patients with neurologic conditions. Pediatr Drugs. 2012;14(4):263–9. https://doi.org/10.2165/11208120-000000000-00000.
22. Mier RJ, Bachrach SJ, Lakin RC, Barker T, Childs J, Moran M. Treatment of sialorrhea with glycopyrrolate: a double-blind, dose-ranging study. Arch Pediatr Adolesc Med. 2000;154(12):1214–8. https://doi.org/10.1001/archpedi.154.12.1214.
23. Zeller RS, Lee HM, Cavanaugh PF, Davidson J. Randomized Phase III evaluation of the efficacy and safety of a novel glycopyrrolate oral solution for the management of chronic severe drooling in children with cerebral palsy or other neurologic conditions. Ther Clin Risk Manag. 2012;8:15–23. https://doi.org/10.2147/TCRM.S26893.
24. Bradford CV, Parman AM, Johnson PN, Miller JL. Pharmacologic management of sialorrhea in neonatal and pediatric patients. J Pediatr Pharmacol Ther. 2024;29(1):6–21. https://doi.org/10.5863/1551-6776-29.1.6.
25. Zanon D, Tumminelli C, Galimberti AMC, Torelli L, Maestro A, Barbi E, Maximova N. Compounded glycopyrrolate is a compelling choice for drooling children: five years of facility experience. Ital J Pediatr. 2021;47(1):222. https://doi.org/10.1186/s13052-021-01173-7.
26. Bachrach SJ, Walter RS, Trzcinski K. Use of glycopyrrolate and other anticholinergic medications for sialorrhea in children with cerebral palsy. Clin Pediatr (Phila). 1998;37(8):485–90. https://doi.org/10.1177/000992289803700805.

27. Reid SM, Westbury C, Guzys AT, Reddihough DS. Anticholinergic medications for reducing drooling in children with developmental disability. Dev Med Child Neurol. 2020;62(3):346–53. https://doi.org/10.1111/dmcn.14350.
28. Lewis DW, Fontana C, Mehallick LK, Everett Y. Transdermal scopolamine for reduction of drooling in developmentally delayed children. Dev Med Child Neurol. 1994;36(6):484–6. https://doi.org/10.1111/j.1469-8749.1994.tb11877.x.
29. Al Jeraisy M, AlFuriah M, AlSaif R, AlKhalifah B, AlOtaibi H, Abolfotouh M. Efficacy of scopolamine transdermal patch in children with sialorrhea in a pediatric tertiary care hospital. BMC Pediatr. 2020;20(1):437. https://doi.org/10.1186/s12887-020-02336-x.
30. Parr JR, Buswell CA, Banerjee K, Fairhurst C, Williams J, O'Hare A, Pennington L. Management of drooling in children: a survey of UK paediatricians' clinical practice. Child Care Health Dev. 2012;38(2):287–91. https://doi.org/10.1111/j.1365-2214.2011.01213.x.
31. Kubba H, Clement A, Grosse S Sialorrhoea (drooling) in children (1187). NHS greater Glasgow and Clyde Paediatric guidelines. 2019. Available at: https://clinicalguidelines.scot.nhs.uk/ggc-paediatric-guidelines/ggc-paediatric-guidelines/ent/sialorrhoea-drooling-in-children-1187. Accessed 15 Oct 2025.
32. Franco JB, Cacita N, Albuquerque Freua KA, Ortega KL, de Melo Peres MPS. Treatment of drooling with scopolamine in pediatric ICU: a case series report. Spec Care Dentist. 2018;38(6):362–6. https://doi.org/10.1111/scd.12326.
33. Jongerius PH, van den Hoogen FJA, van Limbeek J, Gabreëls FJM, van Hulst K, Rotteveel JJ. Effect of botulinum toxin in the treatment of drooling: a controlled clinical trial. Pediatrics. 2004;114(3):620–7. https://doi.org/10.1542/peds.2003-1104-L.
34. Mato A, Limeres J, Tomás I, Muñoz M, Abuín C, Feijoo JF, Diz P. Management of drooling in disabled patients with scopolamine patches. Br J Clin Pharmacol. 2010;69(6):684–8. https://doi.org/10.1111/j.1365-2125.2010.03659.x.
35. Dias BL, Fernandes AR, Maia Filho H. Treatment of drooling with sublingual atropine sulfate in children and adolescents with cerebral palsy. Arq Neuropsiquiatr. 2017;75(5):282–7. https://doi.org/10.1590/0004-282X20170033.
36. Yellepeddi VK, Race JA, McFarland MM, Constance JE, Fanaeian E, Murphy NA. Effectiveness of atropine in managing sialorrhea: a systematic review and meta-analysis. Int J Clin Pharmacol Ther. 2024;62(6):267–77. https://doi.org/10.5414/CP204538.
37. Rapoport A. Sublingual atropine drops for the treatment of pediatric sialorrhea. J Pain Symptom Manag. 2010;40(5):783–8. https://doi.org/10.1016/j.jpainsymman.2010.02.007.
38. Parrott M, Yathavan B, Averin O, Hoggard L, Rower JE, Voight M, Greene D, Tarrell A, Whelan A, Ghandehari H, Murphy N, Yellepeddi V. Clinical pharmacokinetics of atropine oral gel formulation in healthy volunteers. Clin Transl Sci. 2024;17(3):e13753. https://doi.org/10.1111/cts.13753.
39. Petkus KD, Noritz GH, Glader L. Examining the role of sublingual atropine for the treatment of sialorrhea in patients with neurodevelopmental disabilities: a retrospective review. J Clin Med. 2023;12(16):5238. https://doi.org/10.3390/jcm12165238.
40. Norderyd J, Graf J, Marcusson A, Nilsson K, Sjöstrand E, Steinwall G, Ärleskog E, Bågesund M. Sublingual administration of atropine eyedrops in children with excessive drooling—a pilot study. Int J Paediatr Dent. 2017;27(1):22–9. https://doi.org/10.1111/ipd.12219.
41. Azapagasi E, Kendirli T, Perk O, Kutluk TGÖ, Teber S, Çobanoğlu N. Sublingual atropine sulfate use for sialorrhea in pediatric patients. J Pediatr Intensive Care. 2020;9(3):196–200. https://doi.org/10.1055/s-0040-1708552.
42. Malamed SF. Pharmacology. In: Sedation: a guide to patient management. 6th ed. St. Louis: Elsevier; 2018. p. 345–6.
43. Reddihough D, Johnson H, Staples M, Hudson I, Exarchos H. Use of benzhexol hydrochloride to control drooling of children with cerebral palsy. Dev Med Child Neurol. 1990;32(11):985–9. https://doi.org/10.1111/j.1469-8749.1990.tb08121.x.
44. Carranza-del Rio J, Clegg NJ, Moore A, Delgado MR. Use of trihexyphenidyl in children with cerebral palsy. Pediatr Neurol. 2011;44(3):202–6. https://doi.org/10.1016/j.pediatrneurol.2010.09.008.

45. Begbie F, Walker G, Kubba H, Sabharwal A. Acute colonic pseudo-obstruction in a child taking trihexyphenidyl for drooling: prescribers beware. Int J Pediatr Otorhinolaryngol. 2015;79(6):932–4. https://doi.org/10.1016/j.ijporl.2015.03.027.
46. Giess R, Naumann M, Werner E, Riemann R, Beck M, Puls I, Reiners C, Toyka KV. Injections of botulinum toxin a into the salivary glands improve sialorrhoea in amyotrophic lateral sclerosis. J Neurol Neurosurg Psychiatry. 2000;69:121–3. https://doi.org/10.1136/jnnp.69.1.121.
47. Pal PK, Calne DB, Calne S, Tsui JK. Botulinum toxin A as treatment for drooling saliva in PD. Neurology. 2000;54(1):244–7. https://doi.org/10.1212/WNL.54.1.244.
48. Jongerius PH, Rotteveel JJ, van den Hoogen F, Joosten F, van Hulst K, Gabreëls FJM. Botulinum toxin A: a new option for treatment of drooling in children with cerebral palsy. Presentation of a case series. Eur J Pediatr. 2001;160(8):509–12. https://doi.org/10.1007/s004310100784.
49. Suskind DL, Tilton A. Clinical study of botulinum toxin A in the treatment of sialorrhea in children with cerebral palsy. Laryngoscope. 2002;112(1):73–81. https://doi.org/10.1097/00005537-200201000-00014.
50. Bekkers S, Delsing CP, Kok SE, van Hulst K, Erasmus CE, Scheffer ART, van den Hoogen FJA. Randomized controlled trial comparing botulinum vs surgery for drooling in neurodisabilities. Neurology. 2019;92(11):e1195–204. https://doi.org/10.1212/WNL.0000000000007081.
51. Bekkers S, Kok SE, Pruijn IMJ, Delsing CP, van der Burg JJW, van Hulst K, Scheffer ART, van den Hoogen FJA. Surgery versus botulinum neurotoxin A to reduce drooling and improve daily life for children with neurodevelopmental disabilities: a randomized controlled trial. Dev Med Child Neurol. 2021;63(11):1351–9. https://doi.org/10.1111/dmcn.14924.
52. Berweck S, Bonikowski M, Kim H, Althaus M, Flatau-Baqué B, Mueller D, Banach MD. Placebo-controlled trial of incobotulinumtoxinA for sialorrhea in children: SIPEXI. Neurology. 2021;97(14):e1425–36. https://doi.org/10.1212/WNL.0000000000012573.
53. Heikel T, Patel S, Ziai K, Shah SJ, Lighthall JG. Botulinum toxin A in the management of pediatric sialorrhea: a systematic review. Ann Otol Rhinol Laryngol. 2023;132(2):200–6. https://doi.org/10.1177/00034894221078365.
54. Orriëns LB, van Hulst K, van der Burg JJW, van den Hoogen FJA, Willemsen MAAP, Erasmus CE. Comparing the evidence for botulinum neurotoxin injections in paediatric anterior drooling: a scoping review. Eur J Pediatr. 2024;183(1):83–93. https://doi.org/10.1007/s00431-023-05309-1.
55. Oliveira JB, Evêncio-Neto J, Baratella-Evêncio L. Histological and immunohistochemical findings of botulinum toxin action in salivary gland. Braz J Biol. 2017;77(2):251–9. https://doi.org/10.1590/1519-6984.11115.
56. Jost WH, Bäumer T, Laskawi R, Slawek J, Spittau B, Steffen A, Winterholler M, Bavikatte G. Therapy of sialorrhea with botulinum neurotoxin. Neurol Ther. 2019;8(2):273–88. https://doi.org/10.1007/s40120-019-00155-6.
57. Banerjee KJ, Glasson C, O'Flaherty SJ. Parotid and submandibular botulinum toxin A injections for sialorrhoea in children with cerebral palsy. Dev Med Child Neurol. 2006;48(11):883–7. https://doi.org/10.1017/S0012162206001939.
58. Alrefai AH, Aburahma SK, Khader YS. Treatment of sialorrhea in children with cerebral palsy: a double-blind placebo-controlled trial. Clin Neurol Neurosurg. 2009;111(1):79–82. https://doi.org/10.1016/j.clineuro.2008.09.001.
59. Jongerius PH, Rotteveel JJ, van Limbeek J, Gabreëls FJM, van Hulst K, van den Hoogen FJA. Botulinum toxin effect on salivary flow rate in children with cerebral palsy. Neurology. 2004;63(8):1371–5. https://doi.org/10.1212/01.wnl.0000142040.57474.a6.
60. Reddihough DS, Erasmus CE, Johnson H, McKellar GM, Jongerius PH. Botulinum toxin assessment, intervention and aftercare for paediatric and adult drooling: international consensus statement. Eur J Neurol. 2010;17(Suppl 2):109–21. https://doi.org/10.1111/j.1468-1331.2010.03131.x.

61. Wu KPH, Ke JY, Chen CY, Chen CL, Chou MY, Pei YC. Botulinum toxin type A on oral health in treating sialorrhea in children with cerebral palsy. J Child Neurol. 2011;26(7):838–43. https://doi.org/10.1177/0883073810395391.
62. Reid S, Johnstone B, Westbury C, Rawicki B, Reddihough DS. Randomized trial of botulinum toxin injections into the salivary glands to reduce drooling in children with neurological disorders. Dev Med Child Neurol. 2009;50(2):123–8. https://doi.org/10.1111/j.1469-8749.2007.02010.x.
63. Hassin-Baer S, Scheuer E, Buchman AS, Jacobson I, Ben-Zeev B. Botulinum toxin injections for children with excessive drooling. J Child Neurol. 2005;20(2):120–3. https://doi.org/10.1177/08830738050200020701.
64. Khan WU, Campisi P, Nadarajah S, Shakur YA, Khan N, Semenuk D, McCann C, Roske L, McConney-Ellis S, Joseph M, Parra D, Amaral J, John P, Temple M, Connolly B. Botulinum toxin A for treatment of sialorrhea in children: an effective, minimally invasive approach. Arch Otolaryngol Head Neck Surg. 2011;137(4):339–44. https://doi.org/10.1001/archoto.2010.240.
65. Jongerius PH, Joosten F, Hoogen FJA, Gabreëls FJM, Rotteveel JJ. The treatment of drooling by ultrasound-guided intraglandular injections of botulinum toxin type A into the salivary glands. Laryngoscope. 2003;113(1):107–11. https://doi.org/10.1097/00005537-200301000-00020.
66. Savarese R, Diamond M, Elovic E, Millis SR. Intraparotid injection of botulinum toxin A as a treatment to control sialorrhea in children with cerebral palsy. Am J Phys Med Rehabil. 2004;83:304–11. https://doi.org/10.1097/01.phm.0000104680.28335.b9.
67. Rodwell K, Edwards P, Ware RS, Boyd R. Salivary gland botulinum toxin injections for drooling in children with cerebral palsy and neurodevelopmental disability: a systematic review. Dev Med Child Neurol. 2012;54(11):977–87. https://doi.org/10.1111/j.1469-8749.2012.04370.x.
68. Møller E, Pedersen SA, Vinicoff PG, Bardow A, Lykkeaa J, Svendsen P, Bakke M. OnabotulinumtoxinA treatment of drooling in children with cerebral palsy: a prospective, longitudinal open-label study. Toxins. 2015;7(7):2481–93. https://doi.org/10.3390/toxins7072481.
69. Scheffer ART, Erasmus C, van Hulst K, van Limbeek J, Jongerius PH, van den Hoogen FJA. Efficacy and duration of botulinum toxin treatment for drooling in 131 children. Arch Otolaryngol Head Neck Surg. 2010;136(9):873–7. https://doi.org/10.1001/archoto.2010.147.
70. van der Burg JJW, Jongerius PH, van Limbeek J, van Hulst K, Rotteveel JJ. Social interaction and self-esteem of children with cerebral palsy after treatment for severe drooling. Eur J Pediatr. 2006;165(1):37–41. https://doi.org/10.1007/s00431-005-1759-z.
71. van Hulst K, van der Burg JJW, Jongerius PH, Geurts ACH, Erasmus CE. Changes in severity and impact of drooling after submandibular gland botulinum neurotoxin A injections in children with neurodevelopmental disabilities. Dev Med Child Neurol. 2019;62(3):354–62. https://doi.org/10.1111/dmcn.14391.
72. Bekkers S, Leow TYS, Van Hulst K, Orriëns LB, Scheffer ART, Van Den Hoogen FJA. Repeated onabotulinum neurotoxin A injections for drooling in children with neurodisability. Dev Med Child Neurol. 2021;63(8):991–7. https://doi.org/10.1111/dmcn.14872.
73. Carr WW, Jain N, Sublett JW. Immunogenicity of botulinum toxin formulations: potential therapeutic implications. Adv Ther. 2021;38(10):5046–64. https://doi.org/10.1007/s12325-021-01882-9.
74. Hefter H, Hartmann C, Kahlen U, Moll M, Bigalke H. Prospective analysis of neutralising antibody titres in secondary non-responders under continuous treatment with a botulinumtoxin type A preparation free of complexing proteins—a single cohort 4-year follow-up study. BMJ Open. 2012;2(4):e000646. https://doi.org/10.1136/bmjopen-2011-000646.
75. Samadzadeh S, Ürer B, Brauns R, Rosenthal D, Lee J-I, Albrecht P, Hefter H. Clinical implications of difference in antigenicity of different botulinum neurotoxin type A preparations: clinical take-home messages from our research pool and literature. Toxins. 2020;12(8):499. https://doi.org/10.3390/toxins12080499.

76. Nordgarden H, Østerhus I, Møystad A, Asten P, Johnsen ULH, Storhaug K, Løven JØ. Drooling: are botulinum toxin injections into the major salivary glands a good treatment option? J Child Neurol. 2012;27(4):458–64. https://doi.org/10.1177/0883073811419365.
77. Merz Pharmaceuticals, Inc. XEOMIN® (incobotulinumtoxinA) for injection: prescribing information (U.S. FDA Label, Application No. 125360s093). U.S. Department of Health and Human Services, Food and Drug Administration. 2021. Available at: https://www.accessdata.fda.gov/drugsatfda_docs/label/2021/125360s093lbl.pdf. Accessed 15 Dec 2025.
78. Shaari CM, George E, Wu BL, Biller HF, Sanders I. Quantifying the spread of botulinum toxin through muscle fascia. Laryngoscope. 1991;101(9):960–4. https://doi.org/10.1288/00005537-199109000-00006.
79. Shariat-Madar B, Chun RH, Sulman CG, Conley SF. Safety of ultrasound-guided botulinum toxin injections for Sialorrhea as performed by pediatric otolaryngologists. Otolaryngol Head Neck Surg. 2016;154(5):924–7. https://doi.org/10.1177/0194599816629612.
80. Ha TA, Shih MC, Lambert EM. Comparing botulinum toxin and 4-duct ligation for sialorrhea in children — a systematic review. Am J Otolaryngol. 2024;45(2):104119. https://doi.org/10.1016/j.amjoto.2023.104119.
81. Tiigimäe-Saar J, Taba P, Tamme T. Does Botulinum neurotoxin type A treatment for sialorrhea change oral health? Clin Oral Investig. 2017;21(3):795–800. https://doi.org/10.1007/s00784-016-1826-z.
82. Totuk Ö, Kaya E, Sancar EN, Emre SA, Demir S. Iatrogenic botulism after botulinum toxin type A: five cases. Neurol Asia. 2024;29(3):843–7. https://doi.org/10.54029/2024nhi.
83. Öztürk S, Tomruk Sütbeyaz S, Per H. Iatrogenic botulism following botulinum toxin injection in a child with cerebral palsy: a case report. J Child Neurol. (Online ahead of print). 2025; https://doi.org/10.1177/08830738251395996.
84. Gok G, Cox N, Bajwa J, Christodoulou D, Moody A, Howlett DC. Ultrasound-guided injection of botulinum toxin A into the submandibular gland in children and young adults with sialorrhoea. Br J Oral Maxillofac Surg. 2013;51(3):231–3. https://doi.org/10.1016/j.bjoms.2012.07.012.
85. So JI, Song DH, Park JH, Choi E, Yoon JY, Yoo Y, Chung ME. Accuracy of ultrasound-guided and non-ultrasound-guided botulinum toxin injection into cadaver salivary glands. Ann Rehabil Med. 2017;41(1):51–7. https://doi.org/10.5535/arm.2017.41.1.51.
86. Daniel SJ, Schwarz Y. Salivary gland disease in children. In: Flint PW, Haughey BH, Lund VJ, Robbins KT, Thomas JR, Lesperance MM, Francis HW, editors. Cummings otolaryngology: head and neck surgery. 7th ed. Elsevier; 2020. p. 3035–52. https://doi.org/10.1016/B978-0-323-61179-4.00205-2.
87. Lin YC, Shieh JY, Cheng ML, Yang PY. Botulinum toxin type A for control of drooling in Asian patients with cerebral palsy. Neurology. 2008;70(4):316–8. https://doi.org/10.1212/01.wnl.0000300421.38081.7d.
88. Calim OF, Hassouna HNH, Yildirim YS, Dogan R, Ozturan O. Pediatric Sialorrhea: submandibular duct rerouting and intraparotid botulinum toxin A injection with literature review. Ann Otol Rhinol Laryngol. 2019;128(2):104–12. https://doi.org/10.1177/0003489418808305.
89. Calim OF, Polat E, Ozturan O. Staggered botulinum toxin-A injections into parotid and submandibular glands prior to four-duct ligation for pediatric sialorrhea. Eur Arch Otorrinolaringol. 2024;281(4):2043–51. https://doi.org/10.1007/s00405-024-09022-z.

Surgical Management of Drooling in Children

7

Eric Levi

Learning Objectives

- To understand the framework of drooling treatment and how surgery fits in the big picture
- To be aware of the range of direct and indirect surgery for saliva control with their associated risks, benefits and complications
- To be cognisant of the techniques of saliva control surgery

7.1 Introduction

Drooling is a modifiable condition. It is not predictably perfectly curable in every context, but it is a medically and surgically manageable and modifiable condition. As discussed in other parts of this textbook, the management of drooling demands a multidisciplinary and multimodal approach, placing the burden of disease in the overall context of the medical, psychological, social and practical aspects of the whole child and their caregivers [1, 2]. In some situations, drooling is transient and episodic. Therefore, a watchful waiting, non-invasive approach can be taken. In other situations, although drooling can be prolonged and severe, if the overall prognosis of the underlying condition may carry a significant likelihood of improvement with time, then simpler and non-irreversible options of therapy such as speech therapy exercises, dental appliances, medication or botulinum toxin injection can be considered. In other situations, however, drooling may be severe, or may begin as mild, and continue to progressively deteriorate, resulting in significant secondary effects such as aspiration, airway compromise, pulmonary soiling and other

E. Levi (✉)
Consultant Otorhinolaryngologist Head & Neck Surgeon, The Royal Children's Hospital, The University of Melbourne, Melbourne, VIC, Australia
e-mail: Eric@EricLevi.com

J. Saniasiaya (ed.), *An Overview of Drooling in Children*,
https://doi.org/10.1007/978-981-92-1850-9_7

biopsychosocial and practical complications [3, 4]. In these contexts, surgery can and should be considered in the best interest of the child or young person and their families.

The option of surgery for drooling must be placed within the proper framework of a multidisciplinary (Table 7.1) and multimodal approach [5–7]. Not every child with drooling will need surgery. Surgery, like every other treatment modality for drooling, does not carry a 100% success rate. Because of its irreversible nature and associated procedural risks, sialorrhoea surgery needs to be carefully considered. Surgery must be offered for the right indication, in the right patient, with the right technique, at the right time, with the right resources. The art and science of comprehensive saliva control care is in understanding the complications of severe sialorrhea, the trajectory of the child's underlying condition and the specific treatment goals at a particular point in the journey of care [8, 9].

Sialorrhoea therapy in principle should not follow a conveyor-belt-style rigid algorithm for every child. The hallmark of modern medical care is the personalised application of unique treatment plans for individual patients. It may not be appropriate in some situations to go through the motions of trying speech therapy exercises, then trialling a few rounds of different anticholinergics and then trialling botulinum toxin injection before offering surgery. There are times when a child is so debilitated by their severe sialorrhoea that surgery may be considered as an option far earlier than in others. The key is understanding the severity and trajectory of the condition [10–13]. There are some occasions where it is unethical to withhold or delay surgery if the child is in such a severe condition. On the other hand, it may be unethical to offer surgery when the conditions are so severe that any intervention is futile. It is for this reason that we strongly argue for an expert multidisciplinary team approach to include medical, surgical and allied health teams. It is critical to have the medical and allied health representatives in a multidisciplinary saliva control clinic to provide a longitudinal prognostication on the patient's condition so as to better place any surgical intervention in the right timeline of progress.

The goal of sialorrhoea surgery is improvement in quality of life, not curative perfection. Surgery can be performed in stages, keeping in mind that each surgical step is irreversible. The risks of performing surgery need to be weighed against the

Table 7.1 Multidisciplinary Saliva Control Group

Multidisciplinary and multimodal approach to drooling care may involve the following specialties	
General paediatric	Genetics
Neurodevelopmental and disability	Dental surgery
Neurology	Speech pathology
Respiratory medicine	Psychology
Otolaryngology (ENT) head and neck surgery	Complex patient navigator or case coordinator
Paediatric surgery	Occupational therapy
Plastic surgery	Social work
Maxillofacial surgery	Ethics, etc.

risks of not performing surgery (i.e. ongoing complications from the disease). Each surgical technique carries unique risks. Choosing the right surgical technique for the right patient requires clinical intuition, teamwork and experience. One could apply the same surgical technique to different patients and achieve varying results due to the individual patient anatomy, physiology, underlying pathology and neurodisability. In some situations, a multimodal combination of surgery with small dose of medication and speech pathology training may well yield the most optimal outcome for improvement in quality of life.

The options of surgery are broad and generally divided into two groups: direct procedures (Table 7.2) on the saliva glands or their ductal system and adjunctive procedures with indirect effect on saliva control (Table 7.3).

Emphasis needs to be made that the surgical options are broad and must be tailored to the anatomy, physiology, pathology, severity and disability of the child and young person. Some of these surgical options are adjunctive and may be performed if there are other anatomical issues with secondary sialorrhoea effect. For example, if a child was unable to breathe though their nose due to severely obstructed nose or they had severe tonsillar hypertrophy, this would result in a significant open mouth posture and inability to initiate effective swallow, therefore reducing saliva clearance. For this reason, a multidisciplinary approach to the assessment of the patient is critical. The patient's overall posture, craniofacial structures, neck control, oropharyngeal tone, tongue mobility, nasal and oral patency, airway safety, swallow, voice, dental status and Gross Motor Function Classification System level must be taken into account. Sialorrhoea is a modifiable condition, and the goal of treatment is quality of life improvement, not complete cure. The unique pros and cons of different surgical procedures will be discussed in the following section.

7.2 Submandibular Duct Ligation (Fig. 7.1)

7.2.1 Techniques and Tips

1. Transoral approach. In small kids, nasal endotracheal intubation would be recommended to leave more room in the mouth. In older kids, oral ETT taped to the upper lip may be acceptable. Paucity of evidence currently for antibiotic use.

Table 7.2 Direct (primary) saliva control surgery

Submandibular duct ligation
Parotid duct ligation
Four-duct ligation (bilateral submandibular and parotid ducts)
Sublingual gland excision and submandibular duct diversion (rerouting)
Sublingual gland excision and submandibular duct ligation
Submandibular gland excision

Table 7.3 Indirect (secondary) saliva control surgery

Otolaryngology
Adenotonsillectomy
Nasal surgery to improve patency (septoplasty, turbinate reduction surgery, reconstructive rhinoplasty)
Maxillofacial/orthognathic surgery
Maxillary expansion or advancement
Mandibular expansion or advancement
Facial plastic and reconstructive surgery
Stomaplasty/cheiloplasty (improving lip patency with local flaps or tendon transfers)
Facial reanimation surgery

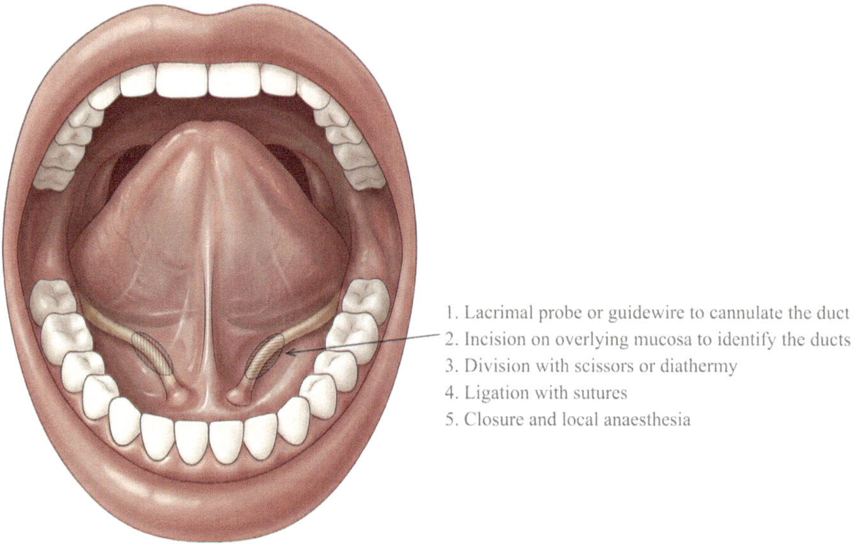

Fig. 7.1 Submandibular duct ligation

2. Cheek retractors, tongue retractor and bite blocks to open the mouth and protect the lips and teeth are used. Stay suture to the tip of tongue for additional retraction can be applied.
3. Lacrimal probe is used to identify the papilla and cannulate the submandibular ducts. A short arterial line guidewire may be a useful alternative. A paediatric 24-gauge cannula may also be an option. Be careful not to traumatise or crush the papilla with forceps.
4. With lacrimal probe in situ, palpation will identify the trajectory of the submandibular duct. Starting about 1 cm away from the papilla, an incision over the duct is made with diathermy or scalpel. The submucosal minor salivary glands and sublingual glands are divided and retracted to expose the submandibular duct.

5. Once circumferential dissection around the duct is done, and then the duct can be cut and ligated with vessel clip, or diathermy and suture. Our institutional preference is suture ligation rather than non-absorbable clips.
6. Closure with dissolving suture (such as 5.0 Monocryl) is carried out, and a small injection of local anaesthesia is performed.

7.2.2 Rationale and Risks

Submandibular duct ligation is a technically straightforward procedure. It is often paired with parotid duct ligation (four-duct ligation) and considered as the least invasive of all the surgical interventions. Applicable to any degree of sialorrhoea and applicable in both anterior or posterior drooling [14, 15]. The ducts may be hard to identify in small patients or in those with micro/retrognathia. If the papilla cannot be cannulated, the ducts can still be identified through the incision with careful dissection. If the dissection is performed meticulously, risks of injury to lingual nerve or blood vessels are low. The rationale behind submandibular duct ligation is to cause obstruction to the submandibular glands and subsequent hypofunction or atrophy of the glands. However, there is limited convincing evidence that this is a truly effective intervention on its own. The anatomy of the duct would suggest that there are multiple perforators into the duct arising from the sublingual glands enveloping the duct. Perhaps therefore there is extravasation of saliva through those perforators in the floor of mouth, and hence there is not a true complete obstruction. There are also anecdotal observations of double duct duplicate anatomy. These multiple perforators and anatomical variations may also explain the lack of reports of submandibular gland swelling associated with submandibular duct ligation. Stone disease in adults often present with pain and swelling associated with calculi obstruction situated more proximal to the hilum of the glands. Perhaps ligation of the ducts distally still allows some degree of extravasation of saliva into the floor of mouth. In short, submandibular duct ligation is a low-risk procedure with a degree of limited evidence of success, approximately 64% based on a meta-analysis [16].

7.3 Parotid Duct Ligation (Fig. 7.2)

7.3.1 Techniques and Tips

1. Transoral approach. Oral endotracheal tube is often sufficient; although in small kids, nasal intubation may provide more room for manoeuvring.
2. Some would use bite blocks to open the mouth, but in our institutional experience, keeping the teeth occluded allows more stretch and mobility around the cheeks. Cheek retractors are essential. Leave teeth in neutral occlusion.

3. Cannulate the papilla with lacrimal probe, arterial line guidewire or paediatric cannula. Once cannulated, use an Allis tissue forceps (or Babcock, Lahey, Mosquito or Arteries) to pinch the papilla with probe in situ.
4. Excise around the papilla to free the papilla and the first 1–2 cm of the duct. The parotid duct differs to the submandibular duct in that it is more adherent in buccopharyngeal fascia and enclosed in the buccinator musculature; hence there is a little more dissection required. The author's preference is the use of fine bipolar dissection in both submandibular and parotid duct exposure. However, any dissection instrument is reasonable.
5. Parotid pain and swelling is a common side effect of parotid duct ligation. To reduce that risk, the author instils transductal intraglandular dexamethasone into the parotid duct with a paediatric cannula immediately before ligation. This is extrapolated from evidence from parotid sialendoscopy. Studies suggest that pain and swelling is reduced when steroid is used as part of sialendoscopy irrigation.
6. Once 2 ml of 8 mg dexamethasone is instilled through the duct, the duct is then ligated with sutures and the papilla amputated. Overlying mucosa is then closed with dissolving sutures and local anaesthesia is injected.

7.3.2 Rationale and Risks

Parotid duct ligation is also a technically straightforward procedure requiring a reasonably short amount of time. Combined with submandibular duct ligation as a four-duct ligation, this procedure is often offered as the first-line surgical therapy as

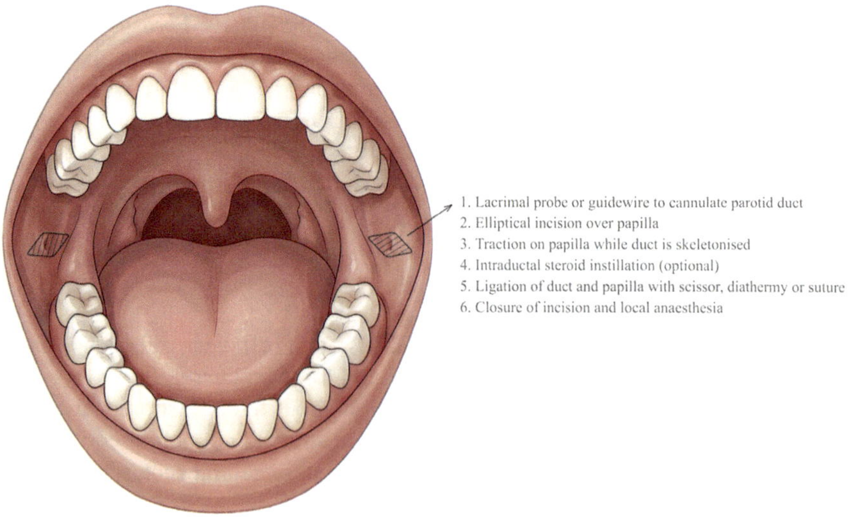

Fig. 7.2 Parotid duct ligation

it does not carry too many risks [14, 15]. Parotid swelling seems to appear more frequently than submandibular swelling for reasons previously discussed (likely more extravasation in submandibular duct and less so in parotid duct). With parotid swelling around the capsule and SMAS layer, pain is more often reported. Hence, to reduce pain and swelling, in the author's institution, the instillation of intraductal dexamethasone prior to ligation is routine practice [17, 18]. Instances of accessory parotid swelling and associated facial swelling have also been described. Of all the surgical interventions, a four-duct ligation has the lowest overall success rate of approximately 64% [16]. In our resource-conscious institution, we are less likely to offer four-duct ligation as we have not found the limited success rate to be acceptable in our patient population. It should be noted that there are anecdotal reports of parotid duct recanalisation with a more proximal fistulous opening. Historically, there have been variations to this procedure including parotid duct diversion and the use of vein graft for duct diversion. These historical procedures have not had strong evidence to support them and are not widely practiced today [19, 20].

7.4 Sublingual Gland Excision (Fig. 7.3)

7.4.1 Technique and Tips

1. Transoral approach. Good exposure is key. Nasal intubation is critical to achieve satisfactory exposure of floor of mouth. Standing at the head of the bed will provide an excellent bimanual approach and ergonomics. Antibiotic is generally recommended as a large exposure of bilateral floor of mouth is expected with resulting dependent cavities once the sublingual glands are excised, although there is absence of studies showing definitive advantage. Cheek protector or retractor, bite block and tongue stay sutures are helpful adjuncts.
2. Begin on one side with a lacrimal probe or arterial line guidewire to cannulate the submandibular duct.
3. Anteroposterior longitudinal incision over the sublingual gland with diathermy (preferred) or scalpel. Begin approximately 1–2 cm behind the papilla. Avoid making incision too lateral or too close to the lingual surface of mandible as the thin mucosa will retract during the procedure, and therefore closure at the end might become difficult.
4. Local anaesthesia might distort the tissue planes, so injecting it at the end may be better.
5. Dissect the mucosa off the superficial surface of sublingual gland. Free the submandibular duct from the sublingual gland. The submandibular duct is enveloped circumferentially by the sublingual gland with multiple microperforators entering the duct. Stay on the capsule of the sublingual gland. Work anterior to posterior to peel the sublingual gland off the mylohyoid base. Long bipolar forceps are good to use here.

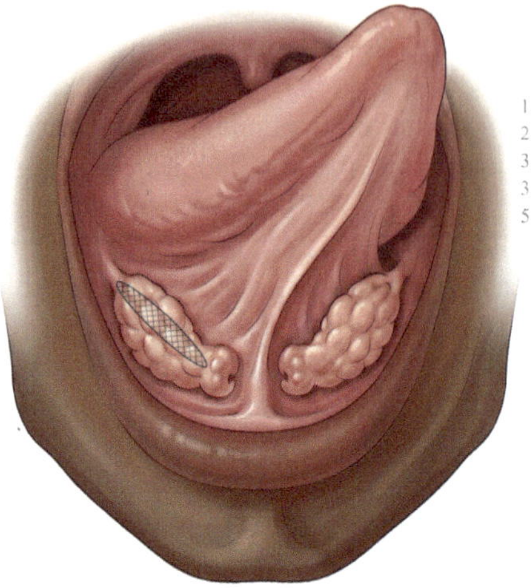

Fig. 7.3 Sublingual gland excision

6. The sublingual gland can extend quite far posteriorly where it abuts the deep portion of the submandibular gland. Care should be taken as injuries to lingual nerve can occur in the more posterior region of dissection.
7. Beware that the lingual nerve and submandibular duct do an intimate rotational twisting from posterior to anterior, so the lingual nerve is quite superficial posteriorly before looping inferomedially as it moves forward.
8. Leave the papilla of the submandibular duct intact and attached to anterior medial mucosa. This allows a good tension as the sublingual gland wrapped around the submandibular duct is dissected free. It also ensures that the papilla remains vascularised and does not atrophy or get unnecessarily traumatised during the procedure. Disconnecting the papilla from medial mucosa too early might result in dry atrophied papilla which will be challenging to secure posteriorly in a duct diversion technique.
9. Once the sublingual gland is freed from the mylohyoid inferiorly, mucosa superficially and the submandibular duct centrally, meticulous haemostasis is to be ensured as floor of mouth haematoma can potentially cause airway emergency or deep neck infection.
10. The next step would be submandibular duct diversion or duct ligation (see next sections).
11. Closure of mucosa with dissolving sutures and infiltration of local anaesthesia.

7.4.2 Rationale and Risks

Sublingual gland excision is a transoral technique that demands a moderate to high degree of technicality. It is almost always combined with submandibular duct ligation or diversion [21]. Postoperative antibiotics and modified diet are recommended although there is a paucity of evidence in this matter. The risk of bleeding or infection to the floor of mouth is higher due to the open exposure, dependent nature of the floor of mouth and continuous muscle movements. Swelling in the floor of mouth may result in airway compromise; hence meticulous intraoperative and postoperative care need to be attended to. Some high-volume centres routinely leave patients intubated overnight to ensure good haemostasis and pain control in the first 24 h [22]. Our institution does not practice routine overnight intubation. We generally extubate the patient at the end of the procedure. Some may require observation in Intensive Care Unit depending on comorbidities. Risk of injury to the lingual nerve is possible in any floor of mouth dissection. Because excision of sublingual gland is routinely coupled with submandibular duct diversion or ligation, we do not have any clear data on the success rate or complication rate of sublingual gland excision alone.

7.5 Submandibular Duct Diversion, Relocation, Rerouting or Transposition (with Sublingual Gland Excision)

7.5.1 Techniques and Tips

1. Following on from steps outlined above, ensure good haemostasis prior to detaching the papilla from anterior mucosa.
2. Create a submucosal tunnel from the posterior aspect of the open incision to the glosso-tonsillar fold or posterior base of tongue. Be mindful that the lingual artery runs deep in the muscle. A small artery forceps, haemostat, mosquito or forceps can be used. Leave a small instrument such as forceps or a small soft silastic suction tube or the smallest nasopharyngeal tube in situ to keep the tunnel patent.
3. Excise a triangular- or diamond-shaped island of mucosa with the duct papilla in the centre. Apply 6.0 nylon, Prolene or PDS on a round tapered needle to each corner. Leave the needle attached to the suture for easier suturing in the base of tongue. Keep the needle and suture protected and individually marked. It would be helpful to know the orientation of the island so as to avoid traumatic twisting during the diversion (Fig. 7.4).
4. Remove the sialstic tube and then deliver each suture through the tunnel that has been created, and exit through the posterior base of tongue opening. Be careful to keep the orientation as much as possible.
5. Once all sutures have been delivered, carefully deliver the papilla and duct through the tunnel (Fig. 7.5).
6. Suture each corner of the papilla island on to the posterior opening, and only then cut the suture needle. This is technically challenging, so a careful retraction of the tongue is necessary.
7. Close the floor of mouth with dissolving sutures. Infiltrate local anaesthesia.

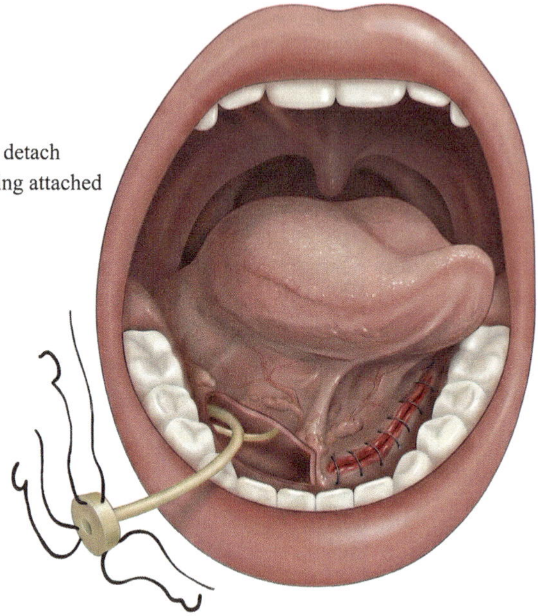

Fig. 7.4 Submandibular duct diversion: mobilising the duct and papilla

7.5.2 Rationale and Risks

Submandibular duct diversion has been a workhorse of salivary control surgery and has been performed for a very long time. Crysdale and his Canadian team has published a longstanding data of nearly 500 children treated with saliva surgery [23]. The procedure of choice between 1978 and 1998 was submandibular duct diversion alone without sublingual gland excision (226 patients). After 1998, sublingual gland excision was routinely included (249 patients). The comparison between the two cohorts revealed that their success rates were similar, but those that had sublingual gland excision had significantly fewer complications, specifically less sialocele, ranula or abscess formation. This would suggest that dissociating the submandibular duct from the sublingual gland potentially causes saliva from the gland to extravasate.

Therefore, submandibular duct diversion along with sublingual gland excision is the recommended surgical procedure nowadays as it is a well-proven technique with a strong evidence base [21, 24, 25]. In the right patient population, it has a success rate of 84.4% [16]. The diversion of saliva flow posteriorly is theorised to stimulate base of tongue activity and increase frequency of swallowing. It also reduces the saliva burden anteriorly and hence very effective for those with anterior drooling or forward posture. There is a reasonable concern of aspiration in posterior droolers. For those with swallowing difficulty, pulmonary compromise and recurrent

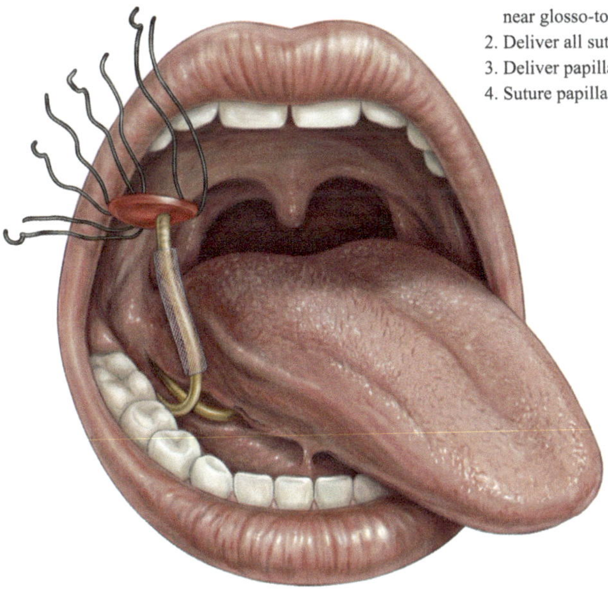

Fig. 7.5 Submandibular duct diversion: submucosal tunnelling

aspiration, submandibular duct diversion is not recommended. It is very effective in anterior droolers, risky in posterior droolers.

However, it is a challenging and time-consuming procedure requiring meticulous technique. There is substantial risk of pain and bleeding from the creation of the submucosal tongue tunnel in addition to the risk of bleeding and swelling from the removal of the sublingual glands. In some centres, patients are routinely intubated for 24 h post-op to avoid primary bleeding or swelling causing airway compromise [22]. In our institution, we routinely extubate patients postoperatively except for a small subset of patients who are very fragile medically. Other potential risks include injury to lingual nerve, delayed bleeding, infection or wound dehiscence.

The diversion or twisting of the duct through the tunnel also places the duct at risk of inadvertent torsion or ligation. A technetium study of submandibular gland function post submandibular duct diversion revealed that not all submandibular glands still worked 3–4 years after diversion [26]. The authors concluded that bilateral submandibular duct diversion maintains long-term function in at least one gland. If the creation of the tunnel and delivery of the diverted duct carries a significant risk of pain and bleeding but only a modest preservation of function, then perhaps a quicker and less risky option such as duct ligation may be a good alternative instead.

7.6 Submandibular Duct Ligation (with Sublingual Excision)

7.6.1 Techniques and Tips

1. Following on from steps of sublingual gland excision, the submandibular duct would have been circumferentially dissected and well exposed almost to its full length.
2. Scissors, diathermy or suture ligation can then be applied close to the posterior aspect proximal to the hilum of submandibular gland (Fig. 7.6).
3. The floor of mouth mucosa is then approximated and closed with dissolving sutures.

7.6.2 Rationale and Risks

Submandibular duct ligation and sublingual gland excision has been popularised by the Italian group in Rome [27]. They call the procedure subtotal functional sialoadenectomy (with addition also of parotid duct ligation) and reported a retrospective cohort of 75 patients surgically treated for drooling with at least 5 years of follow-up. Four-duct ligation (4-DL) was compared with subtotal functional sialoadenectomy (SFS)—which combines 4-DL with bilateral sublingual gland excision. Their study showed that both techniques improved drooling, but SFS produced better long-term outcomes with lower reoperation rates (0% vs ~42% in 4-DL). Complication rates were similar between the two groups [27]. The major concern about submandibular duct diversion is the pain and swelling caused by tunnelling into the base of tongue and potential increased risk of aspiration in posterior droolers with poor swallow. Submandibular duct ligation and sublingual gland excision

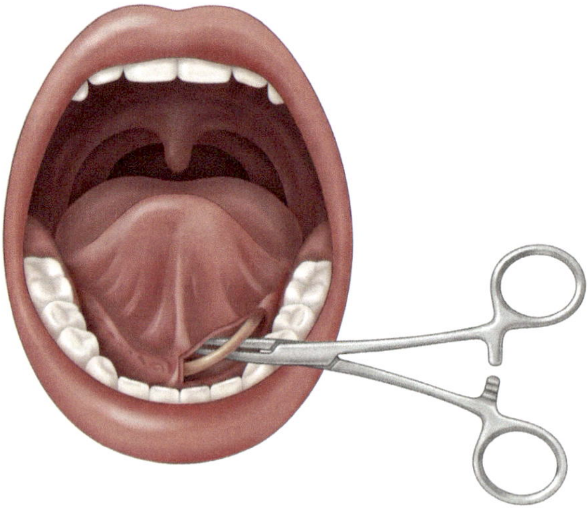

Fig. 7.6 Submandibular duct ligation with sublingual gland excision

circumvents those risks and is therefore a positive alternative as the procedure is quicker, avoids the painful tunnelling of the ducts and has a reduced risk of aspiration. Could this be the one surgery that is applicable to all sialorrhoea patients? A one-size-fits-all solution? Unfortunately, as of today, there is no published RCT comparing SFS versus submandibular duct diversion, so at this moment, there is no definitive recommendation.

7.7 Submandibular Gland Excision (Fig. 7.7)

7.7.1 Techniques and Tips

1. This is a transcervical procedure and technically less demanding than a sublingual gland excision or submandibular duct diversion. The patient is prepped and draped in a sterile fashion to expose bilateral neck.
2. To avoid injury to marginal mandibular nerve, there is a general tradition of using "two finger breadths below the mandible" as a rough guide on placing the incision. It is the author's practice to make an incision on the highest neck crease as it defines the lower border of the submandibular gland and the hyoid bone. This will keep the incision away from the marginal mandibular nerve, provide an acceptable access to submandibular gland and allow for a good aesthetic result.
3. Longitudinal incision on the highest neck crease. Dissect down to the greater cornu of hyoid bone as a reliable landmark for the inferior border of submandibular gland.
4. Subcapsular gland dissection with inferior retraction will avoid injury to marginal mandibular nerve.
5. Facial artery and vein drape the gland's superior and posterior surface sending several perforators that can be sealed with bipolar diathermy.
6. Edge of the mylohyoid is the anterior limit of the dissection.
7. Lingual nerve lies superiorly in a flat V-shaped orientation, and hypoglossal nerve lies deep to the gland just between the anterior and posterior bellies of digastric muscles.
8. Submandibular duct and vascular bundle insert into the gland anteriorly under the cover of mylohyoid. Suture ligation or bipolar dissection is needed to free the submandibular gland.

7.7.2 Rationale and Risks

Submandibular gland excision is safe, predictable and well-tolerated with a success rate of about 85.2%, comparable to submandibular duct diversion [16]. This is the other reliable workhorse of saliva control surgery with an excellent long-term track record [28–31]. Operative time is not prolonged. Most patients will go home on the same day. They will be able to tolerate normal oral intake immediately. This procedure is often offered for patients with posterior drooling for whom a duct diversion

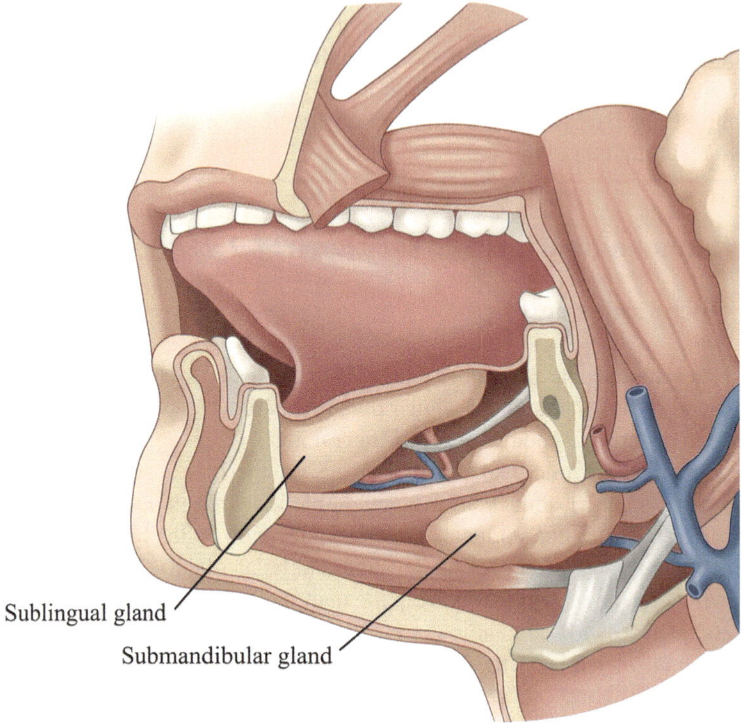

1. Incision on highest neck crease
2. Find greater cornu of hyoid bone as landmark for inferior border of submandibular gland
3. Subcapsular gland dissection
4. Diathermy or suture ligation of duct and vascular bundle

Fig. 7.7 Submandibular gland excision

surgery may be a significant aspiration risk. This procedure is also offered to younger and more severe sialorrhoea patients. Performing any transoral surgery in the floor of the mouth of an infant or toddler is challenging. An open neck procedure would be technically less demanding and for the patient will also stipulate a safer risk profile. This surgery is offered to those patients who are close to, or are already, tracheostomy tube and gastrostomy tube dependent, to reduce the burden of saliva on their airway.

Like any open surgery, the general risk of bleeding and infection is present but low. Risk of injury to marginal mandibular nerve, lingual nerve and hypoglossal nerve can be reduced with meticulous safe surgical steps as outlined above. The concern about visible scar is not something that caregivers are significantly worried about [32]. Placing the incisions on the crease of the neck will provide an aesthetically pleasing outcome (Fig. 7.8).

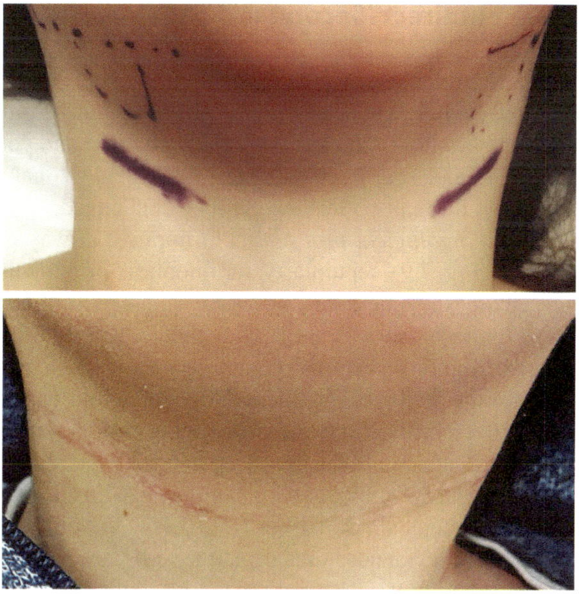

Fig. 7.8 Clinical photograph of bilateral submandibular gland excision scars 7 days postoperatively

7.8 Dental Concerns

Dental caries is always a concern in children undergoing saliva surgery. Causes of dental caries are multifactorial, and dry mouth is one of them. More commonly, cariogenic bacteria, sugar-rich diet, night-time feeding, susceptible tooth enamel and poor routine oral hygiene are implicated. One could have dental caries with normal saliva production, but having dry mouth predisposes kids to increased risk of caries. For this reason, we strongly recommend the presence of a dental specialist as part of the multidisciplinary saliva control clinic. Saliva surgery is offered to children with excessive sialorrhea. Therefore, we commence with a child with excess saliva and poor clearance. The goal of surgery is to improve quality of life by reducing the amount of saliva being produced. Often the anecdotal effects of saliva surgery is a thicker consistency of saliva rather than extreme xerostomia [16, 23, 27, 30, 33]. Removal of some of the major saliva glands still leave the child with thousands of minor salivary glands carpeting the buccal, tongue and oral mucosa. No surgeries are performed to completely eliminate sublingual glands, submandibular glands and the parotid gland function. The goal is reduction, not complete elimination of saliva. To avoid dental caries in saliva control patients, meticulous dental care and carefully staged procedures are carried out. It is not uncommon for us to combine saliva surgery with dental procedures.

7.9 Indirect (Secondary) Saliva Surgery

Saliva control and airway patency are intimately related [34]. The inability to close the lips, occlude top and bottom teeth or breathe through the nose will restrict the ability to swallow and clear saliva. For children and young adults who may already have tone and coordination issues, having additional increased airway resistance will mean that saliva clearance will be challenged.

Otolaryngological procedures to improve airway patency such as adenotonsillectomy (Fig. 7.9), septoplasty, turbinoplasty or other nasal surgeries to improve the airway are, in some cases, necessary adjuncts to the primary saliva control issue. These patients often present with other comorbidities such as obstructive sleep apnoea. Treating the obstructive apnoea will in many situations concurrently improve the saliva management. Not every child with sialorrhoea will require adenotonsillectomy, but adenotonsillectomy will be indispensable for some children with drooling and obstructive sleep apnoea [34].

Maxillofacial or orthognathic procedures are also helpful when there are significant craniofacial abnormalities (Fig. 7.10). Although we do not have large volumes of scientific evidence, first principles and anecdotal reports would suggest that improving craniofacial structures will also improve saliva clearance [35].

7.9.1 Facial Plastic and Reconstructive Surgery

Soft tissue reconstruction to improve lip and oral patency would be a helpful adjunct in the right patient [35]. For example, if a patient had severe facial nerve palsy with resulting droop, saliva dribble and overflow often occur which has negative medical

Fig. 7.9 Tonsillar hypertrophy

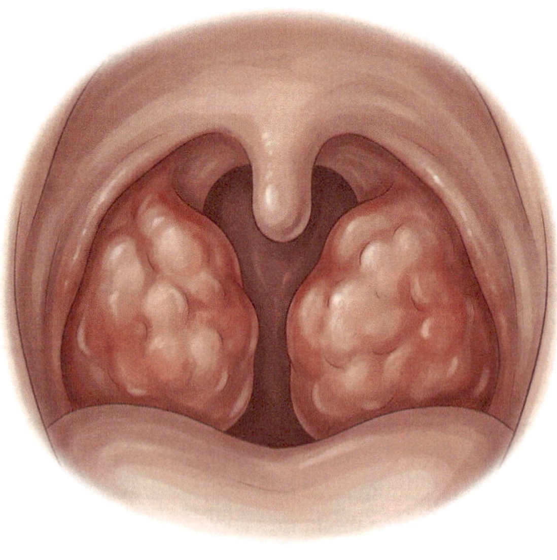

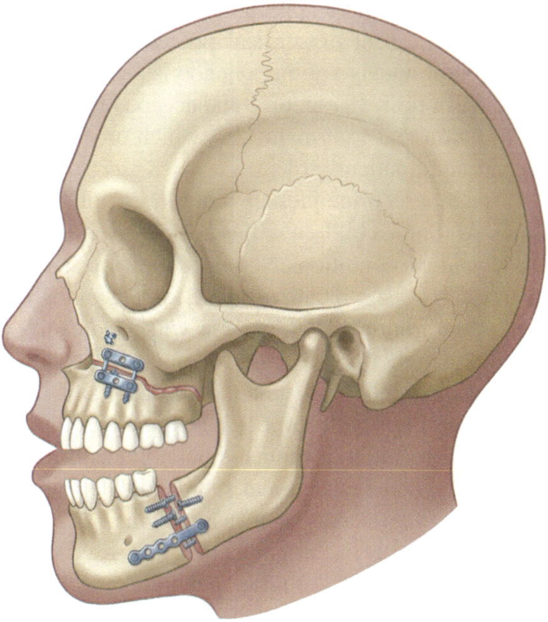

Fig. 7.10 Maxillo-mandibular advancement

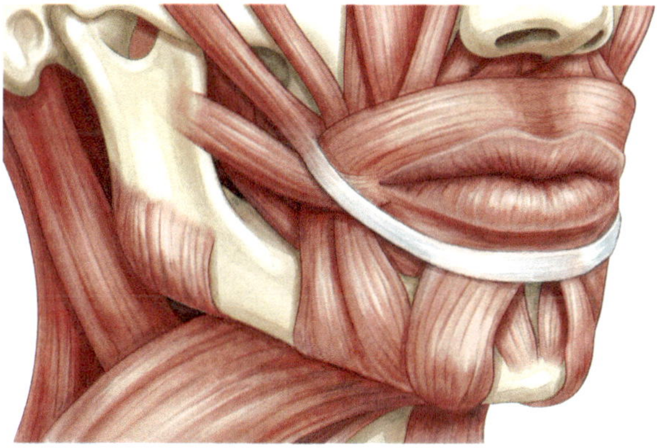

Fig. 7.11 Static sling: palmaris longus tendon transfer to the lower lip

and psychosocial effects. In this case, static and dynamic facial nerve reanimation would improve the patency of the face (Fig. 7.11).

7.10 Which Surgery Is Best?

The answer to this question completely depends on the patient, their comorbidities and their goals of care. Not every child with sialorrhoea will require surgery. There is no single best surgical option that would be perfect for every patient. Some surgeries will be more appropriate for some patients compared to others. We have available a handful of surgical procedures applicable to a very broad group of patients with widely varying phenotypes of their underlying pathology. Every procedure has a positive outcome and acceptable success rate, some better than others. The question that truly matters is which procedure would be most appropriate for that particular patient [36].

Some general principles are worth reiterating again. It is not a conveyor belt trial of therapy. Some children will need surgery earlier than others depending on severity and medical conditions. Surgeries with lower success rates may have lower risks, but also carry a significant resource impact on the health system. A combination of surgery and multimodal treatment with medication and speech therapy is acceptable. In the author's institution for anterior droolers with low risk of aspiration, we would recommend submandibular duct diversion and sublingual gland excision. For posterior droolers with severe disease and high risk of aspiration, we would recommend a combination of submandibular gland excision and parotid duct ligation or a sublingual gland excision and submandibular duct ligation. Multidisciplinary discussion is key. Success is not easily defined as it differs from family to family. For some, a reduction in the number of bibs used per day is sufficient. For others, a reduced frequency of aspiration pneumonia is the goal [36].

7.11 Summary

There is a long list of options for direct and indirect saliva control surgery. Balancing the risks, benefits and timing of every intervention is critical. The big picture matters. Multidisciplinary and multimodal treatment is essential. The goal of therapy is personalised care. Providing the right operation for the right patient for the right indication with the right technique at the right time is the penultimate goal.

References

1. Hughes A, Lambert EM. Drooling and aspiration of saliva. Otolaryngol Clin N Am. 2022;55:1181–94.
2. Reid SM, McCutcheon J, Reddihough DS, Johnson H. Prevalence and predictors of drooling in 7- to 14-year-old children with cerebral palsy: a population study. Dev Med Child Neurol. 2012;54:1032–6.
3. Little SA, Kubba H, Hussain SS. An evidence-based approach to the child who drools saliva. Clin Otolaryngol. 2009;34:236–9.
4. Erasmus C, Van Hulst K, Rotteveel LJR, et al. Drooling in cerebral palsy: hypersalivation or dysfunctional oral motor control? Dev Med Child Neurol. 2009;51:454–9.
5. Daniel SJ, Fayoux P, Bateman N, et al. Comprehensive management of anterior drooling: an international pediatric otolaryngology group (IPOG) consensus statement. Int J Pediatr Otorhinolaryngol. 2023;168:111500.
6. Berweck S, Schwerin A, Heinen F. Management of drooling: 10 years after the consortium on drooling 1990. Dev Med Child Neurol. 2003;45:845. author reply 845–6

7. Daniel SJ. Multidisciplinary management of sialorrhea in children. Laryngoscope. 2012;122(Suppl 4):S67–8.
8. Crysdale WS, McCann C, Roske L, et al. Saliva control issues in the neurologically challenged. A 30 year experience in team management. Int J Pediatr Otorhinolaryngol. 2006;70:519–27.
9. Montgomery J, McCusker S, Lang K, et al. Managing children with sialorrhoea (drooling): experience from the first 301 children in our saliva control clinic. Int J Pediatr Otorhinolaryngol. 2016;85:33–9.
10. Brown AS, Silverman J, Greenberg S, et al. A team approach to drool control in cerebral palsy. Ann Plast Surg. 1985;15:423–30.
11. Sforza E, Onesimo R, Leoni C, et al. Drooling outcome measures in paediatric disability: a systematic review. Eur J Pediatr. 2022;181:2575–92. Outcome measures discussed.
12. Reid SM, Johnson HM, Reddihough DS. The drooling impact scale: a measure of the impact of drooling in children with developmental disabilities. Dev Med Child Neurol. 2010;52:e23–8.
13. Delsing CP, Bekkers S, Erasmus CE, et al. Posterior drooling in children with cerebral palsy and other neurodevelopmental disorders. Dev Med Child Neurol. 2021;63:1093–8.
14. Chanu NP, Sahni JK, Aneja S, Naglot S. Four-duct ligation in children with drooling. Am J Otolaryngol. 2012;33:604–7.
15. Scheffer ART, Bosch KJAM, van Hulst K, van den Hoogen FJA. Salivary duct ligation for anterior and posterior drooling: our experience in twenty-one children. Clin Otolaryngol. 2013;38:425–9.
16. Reed J, Mans CK, Brietzke SE. Surgical management of drooling: a meta-analysis. Arch Otolaryngol Head Neck Surg. 2009;135(9):924–31. https://doi.org/10.1001/archoto.2009.110.
17. Tsikopoulos A, Garefis K, Sidiropoulos K, Triaridis S, Nikolaidis V, Konstantinidis I. Efficacy of sialendoscopy with steroid irrigation for non-lithiasic chronic sialadenitis: a systematic review and proportional meta-analysis. J Clin Med. 2025;14(15):5202.
18. Capaccio P, Torretta S, Di Pasquale D, Rossi V, Pignataro L. The role of interventional sialendoscopy and intraductal steroid therapy in patients with recurrent sine causa sialadenitis: a prospective cross-sectional study. Clin Otolaryngol. 2017;42(1):148–55. https://doi.org/10.1111/coa.12681. Epub 2016 Jun 6.
19. Celet Ozden B, Aydin A, Kuvat SV, et al. Quadruple salivary duct diversion for drooling in cerebral palsy. J Craniofac Surg. 2012;23:738–41.
20. Ozgenel GY, Ozcan M. Bilateral parotid-duct diversion using autologous vein grafts for the management of chronic drooling in cerebral palsy. Br J Plast Surg. 2002;55:490–3.
21. Kok SE, Erasmus CE, van Scheffer ART, et al. Effectiveness of submandibular duct relocation in 91 children with excessive drooling: a prospective cohort study. Clin Otolaryngol. 2018;43:1471–7.
22. Kok SE, Lemson J, van den Hoogen FJA. Postoperative airway management after submandibular duct relocation in 96 drooling children and adolescents. J Clin Med. 2023;12:1473.
23. Crysdale WS, Raveh E, McCann C, Roske L, Kotler A. Management of drooling in individuals with neurodisability: a surgical experience. Dev Med Child Neurol. 2001 Jun;43(6):379–83.
24. Kok SE, van der Burg JJ, van Hulst K, et al. The impact of submandibular duct relocation on drooling and the well being of children with neurodevelopmental disabilities. Int J Pediatr Otorhinolaryngol. 2016;88:173–8.
25. Uppal HS, De R, D'Souza AR, et al. Bilateral submandibular duct relocation for drooling: an evaluation of results for the Birmingham children's hospital. Eur Arch Otorrinolaringol. 2003;260:48–51.
26. Hotaling AJ, Madgy DN, Kuhns LR, Filipek L, Belenky WM. Postoperative technetium scanning in patients with submandibular duct diversion. Arch Otolaryngol Head Neck Surg. 1992;118(12):1331–3.
27. De Peppo F, Caccamo R, Garganese MC, Ceriati E, Marchetti P, Adorisio OD, Cerchiari A, Battaglia S. Subtotal functional sialoadenectomy vs four-duct ligation for the treatment of drooling in neurologically impaired children: long-term follow-up. Clin Otolaryngol. 2021;46(1):222–8.

28. Osorio A, Moreira-Pinto J, Oliveira L, et al. Bilateral submandibulectomy for the treatment of drooling in children with neurological disability. Eur J Pediatr Surg. 2009;19:377–9.
29. Delsing CPA, van den Hoogen FJA, Cillessen E, et al. Bilateral submandibular gland excision for drooling: our experience in twenty-six children and adolescents. Clin Otolaryngol. 2015;40:285–90.
30. Thangirala A, Zhu H, Lambert EM. Submandibular excision with and without parotid duct ligation for sialorrhoea. Br J Oral Maxillofac Surg. 2021;59:1291–5.
31. Delsing CP, Adriaansens C, van Hulst K, et al. Long-term effects of submandibular gland excision on drooling in children with neurodevelopmental disorders: a cross-sectional study. Int J Pediatr Otorhinolaryngol. 2023;164:111377.
32. Delsing CPA, Viergever T, Honings J, van den Hoogen FJA. Bilateral transcervical submandibular gland excision for drooling: a study of the mature scar and long-term effects. Eur J Paediatr Neurol. 2016;20:738–44.
33. Reid SM, Westbury C, Chong D, et al. Long-term impact of saliva control surgery in children with disability. J Plast Reconstr Aesth Surg. 2019;72:1193–7.
34. Kadosh OK, Sever O, Weiss OS, et al. The positive effect of adenotonsillectomy on drooling in children. Otolaryngol Head Neck Surg. 2024;171:554–9.
35. Levi E, Alexander W, Cooper MS. Management of paediatric sialorrhea. Curr Opin Otolaryngol Head Neck Surg. 2024;32(6):444–52.
36. Stamataki S, Behar P, Brodsky L. Surgical management of drooling: clinical and caregiver satisfaction outcomes. Int J Pediatr Otorhinolaryngol. 2008;72:1801–5.

8 Multidisciplinary Approach to the Drooling Child

Rachel Blokland and Shyan Vijayasekaran

8.1 Introduction

Drooling, or sialorrhoea, refers to the involuntary spillage of saliva from the mouth and may be classified as anterior or posterior, or as primary or secondary in aetiology.

While drooling is a normal developmental phenomenon in infants and toddlers, persistence beyond 3–5 years of age is considered abnormal and commonly reflects underlying neurodevelopmental, neuromuscular, structural, or functional impairment [1].

The clinical presentation is heterogeneous, ranging from mild anterior drooling with social consequences to severe posterior drooling associated with aspiration and recurrent respiratory disease [1, 2]. Given the multifactorial nature of drooling and the wide variation in underlying diagnoses, severity, and functional impact, optimal management requires a coordinated, multidisciplinary approach [3, 4].

No single intervention is universally effective, and successful outcomes depend on careful assessment, shared decision-making, and stepwise escalation of therapy tailored to the individual child and family [3, 4].

Multidisciplinary clinics provide an efficient solution to the management of this complex problem in high volume institutions [5].

R. Blokland
Bendigo Health, Bendigo, VIC, Australia
e-mail: RBlokland@bendigohealth.org.au

S. Vijayasekaran (✉)
University of Western Australia, Perth, WA, Australia

Perth Children's Hospital, Nedlands, WA, Australia

Perth ENT Centre, Perth, WA, Australia
e-mail: shyan@perthentcentre.com.au

J. Saniasiaya (ed.), *An Overview of Drooling in Children*,
https://doi.org/10.1007/978-981-92-1850-9_8

8.2 Rationale for a Multidisciplinary Approach

Drooling in children most commonly results from impaired oral motor control and reduced swallow frequency rather than excessive saliva production [6]. Contributing factors may include cerebral palsy, intellectual disability, poor head and trunk control, macroglossia, adenotonsillar hypertrophy, dental disease, malocclusion, sensory processing difficulties, and medication effects [6, 7]. These factors frequently coexist, necessitating input from multiple specialties.

In 2023, the International Paediatric Otolaryngology Group (IPOG) released a consensus statement on the management of anterior drooling, in which it describes a multidisciplinary clinic as being the appropriate approach [3]. A multidisciplinary team (MDT) approach allows for comprehensive assessment of both contributing factors and consequences of drooling, integration of conservative and interventional strategies, avoidance of unnecessary or premature invasive treatments, and alignment of management goals with the child's overall health, function, and quality of life [3, 5]. It also allows for multiple modalities to be utilised in combination [3]. Results of a large case series of 274 children attending a multidisciplinary saliva control clinic suggested that all treatment modalities, including speech therapy, medication, botox, and surgery should be available for effective management of these patients [5].

8.3 Core Members of the Multidisciplinary Team and their Roles

MDT saliva management clinics commonly include input from otolaryngology (ENT), respiratory medicine, gastroenterology, dentistry, occupational therapy, speech and language therapy, neurology, social work, paediatrics, nursing, and physical medicine and rehabilitation, with additional disciplines involved as required [3, 6, 7].

8.3.1 Otolaryngology (ENT)

ENT surgeons play a key role in distinguishing anterior from posterior drooling and in assessing aspiration risk, as well as identifying and managing structural contributors such as adenotonsillar hypertrophy and nasal obstruction. They are responsible for delivering interventional treatments including botulinum toxin injections and surgical procedures when conservative measures fail.

8.3.2 Respiratory Medicine/Pulmonology

Respiratory physicians assess and manage the pulmonary consequences of drooling, particularly in children with posterior drooling and impaired airway protection.

This is important in children with recurrent lower respiratory tract infections, chronic cough, wheeze, or suspected aspiration.

8.3.3 Gastroenterology

Gastroenterologists contribute by evaluating gastrointestinal factors that may exacerbate drooling or increase aspiration risk. Gastro-oesophageal reflux disease (GORD) was shown to be the most common contributing factor (present in 28% of patients) in the case series by Montgomery et al. [5] Assessment may include pH monitoring, impedance studies, or endoscopy where clinically indicated. Optimisation of reflux and feeding strategies can reduce drooling-related morbidity.

8.3.4 Dentistry/Paediatric Dentistry

Dental assessment is essential to identify caries, gingivitis, malocclusion, and oral hygiene issues that may exacerbate drooling or complicate its management. Dentists may also be involved in the design and fitting of oral appliances aimed at improving lip seal and tongue positioning in selected patients.

8.3.5 Occupational Therapy

Occupational therapists address posture, head and trunk control, seating, and sensory processing issues that influence drooling severity. They assist with adaptive strategies to improve daily function and may support behavioural programs aimed at increasing saliva awareness and self-management.

8.3.6 Speech and Language Pathology

Speech and language pathologists (SLPs) are central to both assessment and management. Their role includes evaluation of oral motor skills, swallow frequency, safety of swallow, and risk of aspiration. SLPs provide behavioural and oral motor interventions aimed at improving lip closure, tongue control, sensory awareness, and voluntary swallowing. They also guide decisions regarding the safety of interventions that may redirect saliva posteriorly.

8.3.7 Neurology

Neurologists assist in diagnosing underlying neurological conditions such as cerebral palsy, neuromuscular disease, neurogenetic syndromes, or movement disorders. Neurological input informs prognosis and long-term planning and contributes to medication optimisation, particularly where antiepileptic or antispasticity medications may influence drooling severity.

8.3.8 Paediatrician/Developmental Specialist

The paediatrician plays a central coordinating role, identifying underlying diagnoses, assessing global development, reviewing comorbidities, and ensuring that drooling management aligns with the child's broader medical and developmental needs. Medication review is essential, particularly for agents that may exacerbate drooling or contribute to oral motor dysfunction.

8.3.9 Physical Medicine and Rehabilitation

Specialists in physical medicine and rehabilitation (PM&R) focus on functional optimisation and long-term management. Their role includes addressing posture, tone, and mobility. PM&R physicians often help align oral motor interventions with seating, orthotic, and assistive technology strategies.

8.3.10 Nursing, Social Work, and Caregivers

Nurses and social workers support implementation of care plans, skin care, education, and continuity of care across inpatient, outpatient, school, and community settings.

Caregivers provide insight into the functional and psychosocial impact of drooling, implementing strategies at home and school, and contributing to shared decision-making.

8.4 Multidisciplinary Management Framework

Management should follow a stepwise, MDT-led approach, progressing from conservative to more invasive interventions only when appropriate. The aims are not only to reduce the amount of drooling but also to optimise the child's quality of life and improve self-esteem [8].

8.4.1 Addressing Contributing Factors

Initial management focuses on optimising reversible factors, which may require interventions from multiple specialities. Medications should be reviewed (e.g. paediatrics, neurology), dental problems should be treated (dentistry), and posture should be corrected (e.g. physiotherapy, OT), and if hypertrophy of adenoids and tonsils is present, consider adenotonsillectomy (ENT) [7, 9].

Discouraging excessive oral stimuli (such as mouthing of fingers) with distraction techniques can be tried, but in severe cases may require gloves or elbow splints (OT) [7].

8.4.2 Conservative and Behavioural Interventions

Behavioural measures are usually administered by speech pathologists, physical therapists, or occupational therapists and are aimed at increasing oral muscle tone, stabilising head and jaw position, promoting sensory awareness around the mouth area, and encouraging swallow. The success of such treatments is dependent on the child's level of cognitive function [6].

8.4.3 Pharmacological Management

When conservative strategies are insufficient, anticholinergic medications or botulinum toxin injections may be considered following MDT discussion. Benefits must be weighed against potential side effects, and close monitoring is required.

8.4.4 Surgical Management

Surgical intervention is reserved for children with severe, persistent drooling who have failed adequate trials of conservative and medical therapy. The choice of procedure depends on drooling type, swallow safety, and overall medical status. MDT consensus and thorough family counselling are essential prior to surgery.

8.4.5 Management of Severe Posterior Drooling

In rare cases of intractable posterior drooling with chronic aspiration, definitive airway procedures may be required. This may include tracheostomy and laryngotracheal separation/diversion [10]. These decisions require careful MDT deliberation, involving ENT, respiratory specialists, paediatricians, and the family.

8.4.6 Family-Centred Care and Outcomes

Throughout assessment and management, the MDT must prioritise child- and family-centred care. Goals should include improvements in comfort, social participation, self-esteem, and caregiver burden. Regular review using agreed outcome measures ensures that management remains appropriate as the child grows and their needs evolve.

8.5 Conclusion

Drooling in children is a complex condition with multifactorial causes and highly variable presentation. Parental involvement, understanding family's goals of care, and shared decision-making are essential in this population [3]. A coordinated multidisciplinary approach is needed to achieve safe, effective, and meaningful outcomes. By integrating expertise across medical, surgical, and allied health disciplines, and by actively involving families, clinicians can deliver individualised, evidence-based care that improves both function and quality of life for affected children.

References

1. Lawrence R, Bateman N. Surgical management of the drooling child. Curr Otorhinolaryngol Rep. 2018;6(1):99–106.
2. Evatt M. Oral glycopyrrolate for the treatment of chronic severe drooling caused by neurological disorders in children. Neuropsychiatr Dis Treat. 2011;7:543.
3. Daniel SJ, Fayoux P, Bateman N, Boudewyns A, Brigger M, Chan CY, et al. Comprehensive management of anterior drooling: an International Pediatric Otolaryngology Group (IPOG) consensus statement. Int J Pediatr Otorhinolaryngol. 2023;168:111500.
4. Orriëns LB, De Groot SAF, Van Der Burg JJW, Van Den Hoogen FJA, Van Hulst K, Erasmus CE. Interdisciplinary assessment and treatment of paediatric drooling: two decades of experience by the Nijmegen saliva control team reflected in a stepwise algorithm. Eur J Pediatr. 2024;183(9):3979–85.
5. Montgomery J, McCusker S, Lang K, Grosse S, Mace A, Lumley R, et al. Managing children with sialorrhoea (drooling): experience from the first 301 children in our saliva control clinic. Int J Pediatr Otorhinolaryngol. 2016;85:33–9.
6. Neeraj Mathur. 2022. Drooling (Sialorrhoea). Medscape.
7. Fairhurst CBR, Cockerill H. Management of drooling in children. Arch Dis Child Educ Pract. 2010;96(1):25–30.
8. Van Der Burg JJW, Jongerius PH, Van Limbeek J, Van Hulst K, Rotteveel JJ. Social interaction and self-esteem of children with cerebral palsy after treatment for severe drooling. Eur J Pediatr. 2006;165(1):37–41.
9. The Royal Children's Hospital Melbourne. Saliva control in children: an information guide for families and clinicians. 2017. Available from: https://www.rch.org.au/uploadedfiles/main/content/plastic/salivabook.pdf.
10. Pollaers K, Vijayasekaran S. Surgical treatment of paediatric drooling. In: Open access atlas of otolaryngology, head & neck operative surgery. University of Cape Town; 2020.

Drooling in Developmentally Healthy Children

9

Jeyasakthy Saniasiaya and Graeme van der Meer

9.1 Introduction

Drooling is considered a normal condition in a growing child [1]. It typically persists until 18 months of age and is linked to oromotor control, which is attained between 12 and 16 months. Drooling is generally considered acceptable until the age of 4. It is rarely observed in newborns and becomes evident once infants can maintain their head in a prone position, reported to occur at approximately 2.3 months of age [2].

In an otherwise healthy child, drooling improves with maturation of oral sensory-motor function, which results in progressive refinement and coordination of swallowing [3]. Saliva control therefore represents an important developmental milestone.

Drooling has been reported in approximately 0.6% of the general population [4] and has traditionally been associated with neurological or neuromuscular conditions. However, emerging evidence demonstrates that drooling occurs in otherwise developmentally healthy children [5]. Pathological drooling has been reported in approximately 3% of healthy children, as demonstrated by van Hulst et al. [6] The precise incidence in healthy children remains unknown, in part because drooling is not routinely assessed as a developmental milestone.

J. Saniasiaya (✉)
Department of Otorhinolaryngology, Faculty of Medicine, Universiti Malaya, Kuala Lumpur, Malaysia
e-mail: jeyasakthy@um.edu.my

G. van der Meer
Department of Otorhinolaryngology, Starship Children's Hospital, Auckland, New Zealand
e-mail: graemev@adhb.govt.nz

J. Saniasiaya (ed.), *An Overview of Drooling in Children*,
https://doi.org/10.1007/978-981-92-1850-9_9

9.2 Definitions and Classification

Sialorrhoea (synonymous with ptyalism or hypersalivation) refers to the excessive pooling or loss of saliva beyond the oral cavity. Two anatomically distinct patterns are recognised:

Anterior sialorrhoea describes the forward escape of saliva past the lip commissures onto the chin, face, and clothing. This is the predominant pattern in otherwise healthy drooling children and results from failure to achieve a complete anterior lip seal, often in the context of open-mouth posture [5].

Posterior sialorrhoea describes saliva spilling posteriorly into the pharynx without an adequate swallow trigger. This pattern carries a higher risk of pulmonary aspiration and is more commonly associated with neurological impairment. It is less prevalent in the healthy paediatric population.

9.3 Consequences of Drooling

Unmanaged drooling in otherwise healthy children is not merely a cosmetic or social inconvenience. The consequences span physical, psychological, and developmental domains:

- *Skin maceration and perioral dermatitis*: persistent moisture causes erythema, excoriation, and secondary bacterial or fungal infection around the chin, cheeks, and neck.
- *Dehydration*: daily salivary losses in significant sialorrhoea can exceed physiologically meaningful volumes.
- *Dental complications*: altered salivary flow patterns and pooling contribute to enamel erosion and increased caries susceptibility.
- *Social embarrassment and stigmatisation*: visible drooling is poorly tolerated by peers and can precipitate bullying, social withdrawal, and reduced participation in group activities.
- *Reduced self-esteem*: children who are aware of their drooling may become self-conscious, leading to avoidance of social and academic interactions.
- *Impact on caregivers and family*: frequent clothing changes, bib use, and skin care impose significant practical burdens on parents and caregivers.
- *Impaired oromotor development*: persistent poor lip seal and open-mouth posture may reinforce maladaptive oral habits, potentially affecting speech articulation and feeding.
- *Diagnostic significance*: persistent drooling beyond age 4 may be the first clinical signal of a previously undetected sensory processing disorder or neurodevelopmental condition and warrants formal assessment rather than reassurance alone.

9.4 Pathomechanism

Swallowing saliva involves a complex neuromuscular function encompassing reflexive and voluntary actions, requiring the coordinated activity of approximately 30 muscles and 5 cranial nerves [7]. Throughout development, salivary flow increases, and the growing child adapts through practice and progressive refinement until swallowing becomes largely automatic [8]. Pathological drooling has been attributed to a combination of oromotor dysfunction, sensory processing difficulties, and a failure of coupling between the sensation of oral moisture and the swallow trigger [9].

Drooling in the otherwise healthy child is primarily attributed to a disorder of the oral phase of swallowing. This phase encompasses a preparatory component (tongue and mandibular movements forming a bolus) and a propulsive component (transferring the formed bolus into the oropharynx) [10]. Adequate lip seal and sufficient negative intraoral pressure are prerequisites for efficient bolus propulsion [11]. In healthy drooling children, anterior salivary leakage due to incomplete lip seal predominates over posterior drooling [5].

Contributing factors include mouth breathing (most commonly secondary to adenotonsillar or turbinate hypertrophy), poor head and postural control, malocclusion, tongue-tie, and reduced perioral sensory feedback. Contemporary device use also deserves specific mention: sustained downward gaze when using smartphones, tablets, and gaming devices promotes a flexed head-forward posture that mechanically displaces the mandible and compromises lip seal, aggravating anterior sialorrhoea. As screen exposure in children continues to increase, this positional contributor is increasingly relevant in clinical practice. It is further postulated that poor saliva control in otherwise healthy children may represent the first detectable manifestation of a subclinical sensory processing disorder.

Table 9.1 Aetiology of drooling in the otherwise healthy child

Posture and head control
Forward head posture from sustained device use (smartphones, tablets, gaming)
Generalised low muscle tone
Poor truncal support
Oral motor dysfunction
Poor lip seal
Inadequate bolus formation
Reduced swallow frequency

(continued)

Table 9.1 (continued)

Nasal obstruction/mouth breathing
Adenoid or adenotonsillar hypertrophy
Nasal obstruction
Inferior turbinate hypertrophy
Choanal atresia or stenosis
Deviated nasal septum
Allergic or infantile rhinitis
Dental an occlusal factors
Malocclusion
Teething
Lip tie or tongue-tie
Sensory
Reduced perioral and intraoral sensation
Failure of saliva-to-swallow coupling
Behavioural/habitual
Thumb or digit sucking
Open-mouth resting posture (habitual)
Reflux
Laryngopharyngeal or gastro-oesophageal reflux (reflex hypersalivation)
Unknown

9.5 Aetiology

The aetiology of drooling in the otherwise healthy child is summarised in Table 9.1.

9.6 Evidence on Drooling in Healthy Children

Published literature on drooling in developmentally healthy children, while limited, dates to the early 1980s [12].

Johnson et al. described a cohort of 21 healthy drooling children with a mean age of 4.9 years referred to a dedicated saliva control clinic [1]. Open-mouth posture was the most common aetiological factor identified. Saliva control was achieved at a mean of 5 years after initial clinic attendance, and 80.9% of parents rated the clinic experience positively. In contrast, Crysdale et al. proposed no intervention for healthy drooling children [13].

Talmon et al. advocated unilateral Wharton's duct transposition for healthy drooling children, achieving an 86% success rate in their cohort. The rationale was that redirecting salivary flow to the oropharynx would reduce anterior spillage without disrupting normal swallowing physiology [12].

More recently, van Hulst et al. demonstrated that between 3% and 15% of healthy children, aged 4 years and older continue to drool, with 3% meeting criteria for pathological drooling [6]. Chen et al. identified 22 drooling children with no significant comorbidities, supporting the existence of drooling as an isolated developmental phenomenon in healthy children [14].

9.7 Assessment and Management

Drooling may be the first clinical sign of an underlying neurodevelopmental condition. Equally, it may represent an isolated oromotor immaturity or a correctable structural problem. A systematic, stepwise approach is therefore essential.

9.7.1 Initial Assessment

Assessment should include a structured history (severity, frequency, type of drooling, mouth breathing, postural habits, device use, diet, and any developmental concerns) and a targeted examination (lip seal, tongue posture and tone, nasal airway patency, tonsil and adenoid size, dental occlusion, and perioral sensation).

Drooling severity may be quantified using validated tools such as the Drooling Severity and Frequency Scale (DSFS) or bib count methods [14]. These provide a baseline against which response to treatment can be measured.

9.7.2 Multidisciplinary Management

These children are ideally managed in a dedicated paediatric saliva control multidisciplinary team (MDT) clinic comprising a paediatric ENT surgeon, a paediatric dental specialist, and a speech-language therapist. Where a structural aetiological factor is identified (most commonly adenotonsillar hypertrophy), ENT intervention may be both necessary and sufficient.

Management should proceed in a stepwise fashion:

- *Step 1 Conservative*: Reassurance, posture training, oromotor exercises, biofeedback, and behavioural therapy (cueing for swallowing, lip closure reinforcement). Speech-language therapists design individualised programmes. Attention to device-use habits and head position should be addressed at this stage.
- *Step 2 Pharmacological*: For children with persistent drooling despite conservative management, anticholinergic agents (most commonly glycopyrrolate) may reduce salivary output. Botulinum toxin A injection into the parotid and/or sub-

mandibular glands is an increasingly used option, particularly where surgery is not yet appropriate.

- *Step 3 Surgical*: Reserved for refractory cases. Options include salivary duct ligation, relocation (submandibular duct transposition), and submandibular gland excision. Surgery carries procedural risk and should be considered only after failure of conservative and pharmacological measures.

Developmental Review In any child whose drooling persists despite structured management, referral to a paediatric developmental specialist is recommended to exclude underlying neurodevelopmental pathology that may not yet have been identified.

9.8 Conclusion

Drooling in the otherwise healthy child should not be dismissed as a self-limiting developmental quirk. When persistent beyond the age of 4, it warrants structured assessment and active management through a multidisciplinary framework. The clinician should consider the full aetiological spectrum, including contemporary behavioural factors such as prolonged device use and the associated postural changes that aggravate anterior sialorrhoea. Early identification and targeted intervention can significantly improve the child's comfort, skin integrity, social participation, and self-esteem while reducing the burden on families. Persistent drooling despite initial management should prompt developmental review to exclude underlying neurodevelopmental disorders.

References

1. Johnson H, King J, Reddihough DS. Children with sialorrhoea in the absence of neurological abnormalities. Child Care Health Dev. 2001;27(6):591–602.
2. Carruth BR, Skinner JD. Feeding behaviors and other motor development in healthy children (2–24 months). J Am Coll Nutr. 2002;21(2):88–96.
3. Meningaud JP, Pitak-Arnnop P, Chikhani L, Bertrand JC. Drooling of saliva: a review of the etiology and management options. Oral Surg Oral Med Oral Pathol Oral Radiol Endod. 2006;101(1):48–57.
4. Collins A, Burton A, Fairhurst C. Management of drooling in children with cerebral palsy. Paediatr Child Health. 2020;30:425–9.
5. Saniasiaya J, van der Meer G, Toll EC. Drooling in developmentally normal children: a review. J Laryngol Otol. 2024;138(11):1061–4.
6. van Hulst K, van den Engel-Hoek L, Geurts ACH, et al. Development of the drooling infants and Preschoolers scale (DRIPS) and reference charts for monitoring saliva control in children aged 0–4 years. Infant Behav Dev. 2018;50:247–56.
7. Matsuo K, Palmer JB. Anatomy and physiology of feeding and swallowing: normal and abnormal. Phys Med Rehabil Clin N Am. 2008;19(4):691–707.
8. Sheppard JJ. Using motor learning approaches for treating swallowing and feeding disorders: a review. Lang Speech Hear Serv Sch. 2008;39(2):227–36.

9. Burgmayer S, Jung H. Hypersalivation in severe mental retardation. Int J Rehabil Res. 1983;6(2):193–6.
10. Lespargot A, Langevin MF, Muller S, Guillemont S. Swallowing disturbances associated with drooling in cerebral-palsied children. Dev Med Child Neurol. 1993;35:298–304.
11. Bourdiol P, Mishellany-Dutour A, Peyron MA, Woda A. Tongue-mandible coupling movements during saliva swallowing. J Oral Rehabil. 2014;41(3):199–205.
12. Talmon Y, Podoshin L, Fradis M. The surgical treatment of drooling in healthy children. Int J Pediatr Otorhinolaryngol. 1981;3:55–61.
13. Crysdale WS, McCann C, Roske L, et al. Saliva control issues in the neurologically challenged: a 30-year experience in team management. Int J Pediatr Otorhinolaryngol. 2006;70(3):519–27.
14. Chen T, Daniel SJ. Is bib count an accurate quantitative measure of drooling? Int J Pediatr Otorhinolaryngol. 2021;143:110657.

Current Research and Advances in Addressing Drooling in Children

10

Alan T. Cheng, Mercy E. Jatto, and Jennifer W. Lee

10.1 Introduction

The last 20 years has seen major advances in the management of swallowing disorders. These advances are largely driven by a convergence of greater awareness among clinicians and the public, the better understanding of a variety of disease conditions and the improved medical technology, aiding in diagnosis and treatment. The standardised assessment tools are continuously updated and validated, and this provides a method for bringing researchers together to discuss a common platform.

Drooling (sialorrhoea) can be regarded as a swallowing disorder which can be described as unintentional loss of saliva from the mouth, which occurs naturally in children up to the age of 15–18 months. With advancing age, swallowing in children becomes efficient and better coordinated; hence drooling after the age of 4 years is considered pathologic. However, it may occur or re-present in a child when conditions affecting the safe or effective deglutition process have produced a variety of structural, neurosensory or neuromuscular transpositions which then alter the deglutition process in children.

The swallowing mechanism that prevents pathological conditions from anterior drooling and posterior drooling has already been discussed in the previous chapters. The research that is alluded to in this chapter addresses the subset groups to which enhancing or producing a more effective swallowing mechanism, reversing the drooling symptom. Swallowing is divided into several phases involving potentially

A. T. Cheng (✉)
Department of Paediatric ENT, The Children's Hospital at Westmead, Discipline of Child and Adolescent Health, University of Sydney, Sydney, NSW, Australia
e-mail: alan.cheng@health.nsw.gov.au

M. E. Jatto · J. W. Lee
Department of Paediatric ENT, The Children's Hospital at Westmead, Sydney, NSW, Australia

J. Saniasiaya (ed.), *An Overview of Drooling in Children*,
https://doi.org/10.1007/978-981-92-1850-9_10

hundreds of muscle groups. It relies on the coordination of these neurosensory and neuromuscular receptors at different levels of the deglutition pathway for saliva to safely flow from the oral cavity into the oesophageal passage.

In this chapter, the discussion will focus on the latest research that examines the need for developing platforms that aims to improve communication among researchers on the topic of drooling and its clinical impact on the child and parent/carers. There is a focus on drooling where oral competence is the primary issue, where the oral structures such as the enlarged tongue is the main contributor to drooling and the subject of posterior drooling causing aspiration is more specifically discussed.

10.2 Aetiology

The aetiology of drooling is diverse, affecting a heterogeneous group. Understanding the aetiology of drooling in children is essential for accurate diagnosis and management, as it can be a symptom of underlying neurological, anatomical or developmental conditions.

Conditions causing drooling can be grouped as:

Developmental—Drooling is common in infants and toddlers, and this often resolves before the age of 4 years, at which time they would have developed effective swallowing.

Neurologic Disorders—This encompasses neuromuscular, neurodevelopmental and neurodegenerative disorders. This accounts for majority of the cases of drooling in children. These groups of children often suffer from muscular hypotonia, abnormal posture and balance, central neurologic damage and atypical oral sensory processing, all of which results in ineffective, infrequent and poorly coordinated swallowing. The most common disorder in this group is cerebral palsy, which affect an estimated 1–5 per 1000 live births. Cerebral palsy (CP) encompasses a group of disorders caused by non-progressive permanent damage to the developing brain, occurring before, during or shortly after birth, causing abnormal muscle tone, movement and balance, with varying degree of severity in affected individuals.

Anatomic and Structural Causes—Certain structural abnormalities affecting the oral cavity and pharynx are associated with drooling. Macroglossia, cleft lip, dental malocclusion, palatal abnormalities, obstructive adenotonsillar enlargement and nasal obstruction are such examples. They are rarely the sole cause of sialorrhea but often exacerbate underlying conditions. For instance, macroglossia can worsen oral incompetence leading to salivary spillage, whilst midfacial development issues such as Treacher Collins syndrome forces the child to mouth breathe constantly. Persistent mouth opening due to nasal obstruction, malocclusion or other orthodontic abnormalities may further contribute to oral incompetence.

Medical Conditions—Infective or inflammatory conditions affect the oral cavity and pharynx causing drooling, such as tonsillitis and pharyngitis. It may occur as a side effect of certain medications which stimulate hypersalivation such as clozapine and clonazepam among others. Drooling associated with these medical conditions is often acute and reversible with treatment of the underlying condition or withdrawal of the offending medication.

10.3 Assessment

A holistic and structured assessment is essential for guiding the management of drooling in children. A comprehensive evaluation of the swallowing function comes from a proper anamnestic assessment as to the onset of drooling, when is it most severe and how it applies whilst eating, sleeping or at rest. The examination may require a full otolaryngology assessment, with particular inspection of the nasal cavity, the oropharyngeal soft tissues, the size and position of the tongue, the dentition, the velopharyngeal airspace and the collapsibility of the tissues. Ideally, drooling evaluation should be conducted in a multidisciplinary setting, consisting primarily of paediatrician, speech pathologist, otorhinolaryngologist, dentist, occupational therapist, physiotherapist and social worker [1–4].

Subjective and objective drooling assessment tools are utilized in classification (anterior, posterior or a combination), severity grading, quantification of the impact of drooling on the quality of life of both the patient and their caregivers, guiding treatment plans, and evaluating the outcome/effect of treatment [3–6]. Recent researches have clearly demonstrated the importance of distinguishing between anterior and posterior drooling, as they are distinct clinical entities with different impacts and differing morbidities. Posterior drooling is estimated to affect 10–15% of children with central neurologic disorder [7]. Traditional drooling assessment tools such as 5-min Drooling Quotient (DQ5), Drooling Severity and Frequency Scale (DSFS), Bib count and Modified Teacher Drool Scale (mTDS) in children are primarily focused on anterior drooling, potentially leading to underdiagnosis of posterior drooling, which is more strongly associated with significant respiratory morbidity; early diagnosis and intervention is important in prevention of saliva aspiration and its attendant sequelae [7, 5].

In many instances, posterior drooling may be missed by clinicians due to subtle clinical presentation such as frequent swallowing, vomiting and gurgling breath sounds, which may not be linked to saliva aspiration, as observed in a recent qualitative research involving caregivers. This brings to the fore the importance of caregiver observation in the diagnosis of posterior drooling.

More recently greater attention is being given to the development of assessment tools for posterior drooling in children, most of which are still in the process of validation. One of such was developed by Hughes and Lambert [8], where assessment was based on the presence or absence of cough and ch1921oking in different positions (lying, sitting) and also on history of number of chest infection over a 12-month period. Scores of 0–4 were assigned based on findings, with higher scores denoting worse saliva aspiration. Paediatric Posterior Drooling Scale (PPDS) is another such tool, which utilized cervical auscultation to assess the frequency of swallow and the quality of breath sounds pre and post swallow. The result was on a scale of 0–4, with scores of 2 and above suggestive of saliva aspiration. The PPDS was found to correlate to the Functional Oral Intake Scale (FOIS) and the Eating and Drinking Classification System (EDACS) which are scales used to assess children with swallowing disorders with nasogastric tubes and swallowing in children with cerebral palsy respectively [9, 10] (Table 10.1).

Current evidence supports the combined use of subjective and objective assessment tools. Videofluoroscopic swallow studies (VFSS) is considered the gold standard for objective evaluation of the oral and pharyngeal phases of swallowing. It is particularly valuable in individuals with severe or persistent drooling, suspected posterior drooling and recurrent respiratory infections, or when invasive treatments such as botulinum toxin injections or surgery are being considered; additionally it aids in the trial of certain compensatory strategies such as thickeners [11]. Some of the drawbacks of VF is radiation exposure and the fact that saliva is not visible on X-ray, because it does not mix with the radiopaque contrast used in the study [1].

Another comparable examination is fibreoptic endoscopic evaluation of swallowing (FEES), which allows direct visualisation of the pharynx and larynx with swallowing in an awake patient, assessing for pharyngeal residue, saliva pooling and penetration of aspiration of saliva [12]. It has the advantage of no radiation exposure and can be repeated if needed. The development of a pharyngeal residue severity score which began at Yale University by Neubauer et al. [13] has since seen a plethora of similar rating scales in different countries/areas. By classifying residue as none, trace, mild, moderate or severe, the scale helps clinicians pinpoint the underlying physiological causes of dysphagia. For example, high residue levels in the vallecula may indicate tongue base retraction deficits, while pyriform sinus residue often suggests pharyngeal constrictor impairment, leading to specific, targeted interventions. The quantified data (percentage of filling and anatomical location) allows speech pathologists to make informed decisions with respect to compensatory strategies (e.g. chin tuck, supraglottic swallow) or dietary adjustments (e.g. thickening liquids, softened food) to reduce risk of posterior drooling or aspiration. The senior author has also investigated the role of laser dividing the pharyngoepiglottic fold with noted successful improvements to the select patients with clinically significant issues.

Table 10.1 Paediatric posterior drooling scale uses cervical auscultation to assess the breath and swallowing sounds after feeding

Paediatric posterior drooling scale			
0	Clear breath	Saliva swallow	Clear breath
1	Wet breath	Saliva swallow	Clear breath
2	Clear breath	Saliva swallow	Wet breath
3	Wet breath	Saliva swallow	Wet breath
4	Wet breath	No saliva swallow	Wet breath

The scoring of Grade 0 being no posterior drooling and Grade 1–4 the presence and severity of posterior drooling

With advancements in medical imaging and endoscopy, these assessment tools are increasingly more precise in diagnosis and treatment evaluation. However systematic reviews using the COSMIN (COnsensus-based Standards for the Selection of health Measurement INstruments) methodology highlight that no single assessment tool sufficiently captures all aspects of drooling [14, 15]. Consequently, a multidisciplinary assessment is recommended, combining medical history, oral-motor and postural evaluations, caregiver-reported impact and targeted tools for assessing both anterior and posterior drooling. It is important to emphasise the need to have a tool that combines quantitative methods and parent-/patient-reported subjective outcome measures that reports drooling severity and its relevance in a score that reflects the true nature of drooling and its impact. This tool must be assessed in different patient population in different ethnic groups. This comprehensive approach can then explicitly link assessment findings to individualised management pathways which provide clinician/speech pathology confidence in their evaluation, support the clinical decision-making, enhance efficacy of follow-up reviews after therapy is provided and improve on research quality.

10.3.1 Facial Nerve Paresis and Paediatric Drooling

Facial nerve palsy (FNP) refers to weakness or paralysis of the muscles innervated by the facial nerve and may be congenital or acquired and unilateral or bilateral. Facial palsy is the most common cranial neuropathy in children, affecting 21 cases per 100,000 children per year. FNP is 2–4 times less prevalent in the paediatric population than in adults [16].

Causes of FNP include congenital palsy (birth trauma, syndromic or developmental anomaly), Bell's palsy (idiopathic), infection (otitis media, viral, Lyme disease), trauma (including iatrogenic) and neoplastic. FNP can have profound functional, aesthetic and psychosocial consequences for the child and family. Drooling and swallowing difficulty can occur in FNP, in addition to ocular dysfunction, loss of emotional and facial expression and issues with speech and articulation.

10.3.1.1 Pathophysiology

The facial nerve contributes to the oral and oropharyngeal phases of swallowing via motor innervation of the orbicularis oris, zygomaticus, buccinator, posterior belly of digastric and stylohyoid muscles. It also provides innervation to the salivary glands and taste sensation to the anterior two-thirds of the tongue. Patients with injury to the facial nerve generally present initially with flaccid facial paralysis, but through recovery or repair, there is postparalytic facial palsy (PPFP), when synkinesis and hypertonicity may occur, leading to a change in how the FNP can affect perioral function. Flaccid and synkinetic FNP are distinct conditions, requiring different treatment paradigms. PPFP can encompass the full spectrum of facial movement disorders from persistent complete palsy to full return of function and zonal permutations of hypo- and hyperactivity.

Drooling and swallowing difficulty can be a debilitating functional consequence of facial palsy, and the pathophysiology includes the loss of lip elevation due to weakness of the zygomaticus and levator labii and inferior malpositioning of the oral commissure. Patients experience oral incompetence and impaired lip seal, primarily due to weakness of orbicularis oris, leading to anterior loss of saliva. In addition, there is impaired intraoral bolus manipulation and retention of food and saliva in the lower gingivobuccal sulcus due to buccinator weakness. Some children will exhibit lip and buccal mucosa biting due to loss of lower lip depression from weakness of the depressor labii inferioris. When there is synkinesis, the patients experience facial tension and involuntary oral movements which further affect bolus control and patency of the oral commissure. If there is concurrent impairment of trigeminal nerve function, there is reduced facial sensation and awareness of drooling.

A study [17] conducted in 65 adults found that patients with flaccid FNP reported worse oral function, including food and drink spillage, food trapping in the buccal cavity, cheek biting and inability to drink out of a cup, compared to patients with synkinetic FNP. In another study of 27 adult patients with unilateral FNP, 12 patients (46%) reported a specific problem with drooling [18].

10.3.1.2 Assessment

A thorough understanding of how facial palsy affects each patient is imperative. Assessment begins with the history of the FNP with particular attention to chronicity, cause, treatment to date and functional concerns regarding oral competence, food bolus manipulation, nasal patency and speech articulation. The identification of individual goals and expectations are crucial for establishing rapport and tailoring treatment options. It is also imperative to explore the psychosocial concerns of the patient in FNP, including self-consciousness, social withdrawal, depression and anxiety.

Physical examination should focus on zonal assessment of resting facial tone, weakness of volitional movement and presence of synkinesis, comparing both sides of the face. For oral function, assessment should document positioning, movement and symmetry in the midface, nasolabial fold region, oral commissure and lower lip. If surgical facial reanimation is considered, clinical assessment of the function of the nerve to masseter and hypoglossal and accessory nerves is required to assess for suitability as donor nerves and can be supplemented with electromyography (EMG).

Several scoring systems exist for facial palsy, the most commonly used being the House-Brackmann Score and Sunnybrook Facial Grading System. There are also a number of patient-reported outcome measures applicable to FNP including the Facial Disability Index (FDI). Serial photographs, pre- and post-treatment, can help with tracking outcome measures.

The use of investigations is dictated by the clinical presentation of the patient. To identify the cause of FNP, and for surgical planning, investigations may include audiology, MRI or CT imaging, autoimmune markers and viral serology. Electrophysiology is often utilised in assessment of acute facial paralysis and recovery, including electroneuronography (ENoG) and EMG.

10.3.1.3 Management

Whilst there is robust literature describing techniques addressing smile aesthetics for FNP patients, there is significantly less focus on functional perioral restoration. A systematic review in 2021 [19] of oral incompetence arising from FNP found a lack of consistency in the measurement and management of FNP. Further to this, literature around paediatric FNP is even more scarce.

Management of children with FNP requires multidisciplinary input and treatment tailored to the individual patient with aims of achieving symmetry, restoration of function and minimisation of synkinesis. The paediatric patient usually has more favourable resting tone and better neuroplasticity, but the anatomy can be challenging, and craniofacial growth can be a confounding factor to consider. Furthermore, there can be variable patient participation in treatment planning and rehabilitation, particularly in younger age. Age-appropriate education about the patient's facial function, treatment goals and rehabilitation needs is essential.

The components of facial rehabilitation include soft tissue mobilisation, neuromuscular retraining to improve oral competence and synkinesis management. Drooling in patients with FNP is best managed using a multimodality approach including oromotor physical and speech therapy, pharmacotherapy including selective chemodenervation with botulinum toxin and surgery.

Some compensatory strategies for FNP used in oromotor and speech therapy include:

(i) Neuromuscular retraining and strengthening exercises for lips and cheeks, focussing on improving lip closure and bolus control.
(ii) Maintaining good posture and keeping the head upright.
(iii) Massage and taping to support the cheek and oral commissure.
(iv) Sipping water and reminders to swallow more frequently.
(v) Dab rather than wipe the child's mouth and chin.
(vi) Avoidance of sweet and acidic foods which increase saliva production.
(vii) Biofeedback and helping child to become more aware when their face is wet.
(viii) Pharmacotherapy for drooling in FNP includes anticholinergic medications such as glycopyrrolate and scopolamine to reduce salivary secretion. They can lead to dry mouth which predisposes the child to oral candidiasis, dental decay and swallowing difficulties. Botulinum toxin injections can be performed into the parotid and submandibular glands to reduce saliva production. Botulinum toxin is also used in FNP in the management of synkinesis and to improve facial symmetry by chemodenervation of overactive muscles. This reduces mass movement in the affected face and reduces compensatory hyperactivity of the contralateral face. Chemodenervation in the perioral region is often performed to the affected depressor anguli oris (DAO), buccinator, mentalis and platysma to control synkinesis. It is also used in the contralateral depressor labii inferioris (DLI) to improve lower lip symmetry.

In refractory cases, surgery may be indicated in management of drooling in FNP. Salivary duct relocation or ligation and salivary gland excision can be effective at reducing salivary secretion or direct saliva posteriorly [20].

10.3.1.4 Facial Reanimation

Facial reanimation surgery is divided into static and dynamic options. Particularly in the paediatric population, there has been a shift in attention away from static reposition techniques toward dynamic reanimation through nerve and free muscle transfers. The factors affecting decision-making for facial reanimation surgery include the aetiology of FNP, anatomical site of nerve defect, laterality, duration of the FNP and age of the patient.

Multivector fascia lata static slings to the midface and oral commissure restore resting symmetry in the perioral region in the flaccid face by providing suspension and stabilisation. A static sling suspension can be considered during the waiting period for potential facial nerve recovery, or can be paired with a dynamic procedure. Fascia lata is harvested from the lateral thigh, 10 cm superior to the femoral condyle and 4 cm anterior to the lateral intermuscular septum. The fascia lata is then divided into separate bands placed at the modiolus of orbicularis oris at the oral commissure, philtrum, nasolabial fold and cartilage of the nasal ala through a preauricular incision and sub-superficial musculoaponeurotic system (SMAS) dissection. The sling is secured proximally to the temporalis fascia, periosteum of the zygomatic arch or mandibular condyle.

Dynamic options for the mid and lower zones of the face include nerve repair, grafting and transfer, regional muscle transfer and free functional muscle transfer. Nerve grafting and transfers can be considered in the acute to subacute period after facial nerve injury with intact distal facial nerve stump and viable motor endplates. The most frequently used nerve transfers for the perioral region include the nerve to masseter branch of trigeminal nerve and partial hypoglossal nerve, which are coapted to distal branches of the facial nerve.

Regional muscle transfer, of which the lengthening temporalis myoplasty is most common, is suitable if the patient is not a candidate for neurotisation, such as in congenital or chronic FNP. The temporalis muscle is mobilised, rotated downwards on its neurovascular supply and tensioned in a new vector of pull for the ipsilateral oral commissure. The procedure is relatively simple and quick, but disadvantages include lack of spontaneity, increased midfacial bulk and hollowing over the temporal fossa.

The gold standard for facial reanimation in congenital or chronic FNP is free functional muscle transfer, and an active spontaneous smile can often be achieved. The options for donor muscle include the gracilis, latissimus dorsi and pectoralis minor. The gracilis muscle transfer is the most favoured with the advantage of having predictable anatomy, easy access and low donor-site morbidity. The gracilis muscle is harvested from the contralateral leg with its branch of the obturator nerve, and its vascular supply is anastomised to the facial vessels. The masseteric branch of the trigeminal nerve is the most popular choice for source of neurotisation, due to it being a single-stage procedure, purely motor input, straightforward anatomy and dissection and powerful re-innervation compared to a cross-facial nerve graft. Several studies Hadlock et al [21], Harrison [22], Ueda et al [23], have reported lower failure rates and better outcomes of gracilis transfers in children than in adults, with 83–95% complete muscle re-innervation rate, earlier time to movement, good or excellent symmetry at rest and acceptable spontaneity of smile. Importantly, the gracilis flap will grow synchronously with the craniofacial skeleton. The optimal timing for proceeding with free muscle transfer is debatable, with most surgeons recommending intervention after 6 years of age so that the child can be self-aware and mature enough to understand and participate in decision-making and rehabilitation requirements.

Postoperative rehabilitation is required to maximise the potential for re-innervation and muscle function and must be age-appropriate for paediatric patients. Rehabilitation includes initial stretching and facial massage to prevent scarring and maintain muscle pliability, followed by neuromuscular retraining and feedback therapy. When nerve to masseter is used as the donor nerve, rehabilitation involves training the patient to bite and activate the masseter. When hypoglossal reconstruction is performed, therapy is focussed on controlling tongue placement and movement.

Surgical management of synkinesis may include selective neurolysis or myectomy, after a trial of botulinum chemodenervation and/or local anaesthetic. Myectomy may be indicated for the affected DAO to increase commissure excursion and smile angle, or contralateral DLI to reduce downward pull of the lower lip.

10.3.2 Macroglossia and Drooling

It is now recognised that relative macroglossia may contribute to the inability to achieve appropriate upper and lower lip competence, hence predisposing the patient to chronic anterior drooling. The tongue and its posterior position in the oropharynx may potentially allow spillover of oral secretions straight into the supraglottic airway, predisposing to posterior drooling in certain head positions. It is well-known that should there be an acute inflammatory condition, the size of the tongue and its position will cause tongue protrusion, respiratory distress and dysphagia. However, there is an increasing awareness that the prevalence of chronic relative macroglossia do occur, and increasing case reports into its management is now described [24].

Beckwith-Wiedemann Syndrome is a human genomic imprinting disorder of chromosome 11p15.5 region, which causes epigenetic defects. Its phenotypic variability can produce tissue overgrowth, macroglossia, abdominal wall defects, lateralised overgrowth and a predisposition to embryonal tumours. What is now recognised is that there is a Beckwith-Wiedemann spectrum disorder, which is the most common cause of macroglossia in childhood, and up to 40% of cases do require surgical tongue reduction [25]. The indications for intervention include difficulty with feeding, persistent drooling, articulation issues, orthodontic problems, the development of prognathism and an anterior open bite deformity. As demonstrated in the international consensus documents on Beckwith-Wiedemann syndrome [26], if there is airway obstruction, careful evaluation by respiratory/sleep physicians and an otolaryngologist is necessary, and tongue reduction should be considered after the age of 1 year old, if there are macroglossia-associated feeding problems, persistent drooling, speech difficulties, dental malocclusion and psycho-social problems caused by the altered appearance. Tongue reduction surgery should be performed by an experienced surgical team after detailed assessment by a multi-disciplinary team (including paediatric anaesthesiologists, intensive care unit members, surgeons, speech therapists and orthodontists), preferably in a reference centre, and the results should be carefully audited, and postoperative follow-up should continue until the age of 16 years.

Discussion on the types of tongue reduction surgery can be found in reference articles such as Chau et al. [27] who describes the procedure as follows: "This can be performed using a mouth retractor without a tongue blade and silk traction sutures to assist tongue retraction. An inverted V incision through the tongue surface and musculature is carried out using electrocautery, CO2 laser or a 'cold steel' surgical blade. The incision is bevelled, cutting toward deep musculature, in order to have more mucosal surface to reapproximate and to decrease tension on the suture line. The tongue is closed in layers using absorbable sutures to reapproximate the tongue musculature (2/0 Polydioxanone suture (PDS)) and the mucosal surfaces (4/0 vicryl)" (Fig. 10.1).

The literature divides the types of surgical techniques from tip amputations, anterior wedge resection, central reductions, dorsal flap excisions, marginal excisions and combination procedures. The aim is to maintain the inferolateral neuromuscular bundles, but the goal is to restore the shape and size and function of the tongue and correct the functional abnormalities of drooling, achieving lip closure; maintain taste and mobility function; improve breathing outcomes; and correct obstructed sleep disordered breathing. The feeding outcomes were summarised by Abraha et al. [28] noting significant improvements in drooling, decreased spillage of food and fluid due to reduced tongue protrusion, significant improvement in biting, lip seal, and bolus manipulation, mild residual difficulties in biting, tongue lateralisation, and bolus manipulation 3 months post-operatively. Shipster et al. [29] also reported specifically drooling was significantly decreased and ceased in all but one patient 1 year after surgery. However, in all the studies examined, there is still debate on the exact timing of surgery and complexity in determining indications and outcome measures.

The other subgroups with relative macroglossia include children with Trisomy 21 and Klippel-Trenaunay-Weber syndrome and children with oral lymphatic malformations. Arslan et al. [30] in their study comparing Trisomy 21 children with normal developing children and using the Pediatric version of the Eating Assessment Tool-10 (PEDI EAT-10) confirmed the significant statistical difference in rates of drooling (31.3%) in Trisomy 21 children as compared to the controls, as well as the higher rates of coughing with normal swallowing (41.7%). Tongue reduction in Trisomy 21 children is well described, and feeding outcomes and drooling resolution herald back to Starmans et al. [31]. Posterior tongue base reduction requires resection of a rhomboid wedge of midline tongue tissue, which assists in debulking

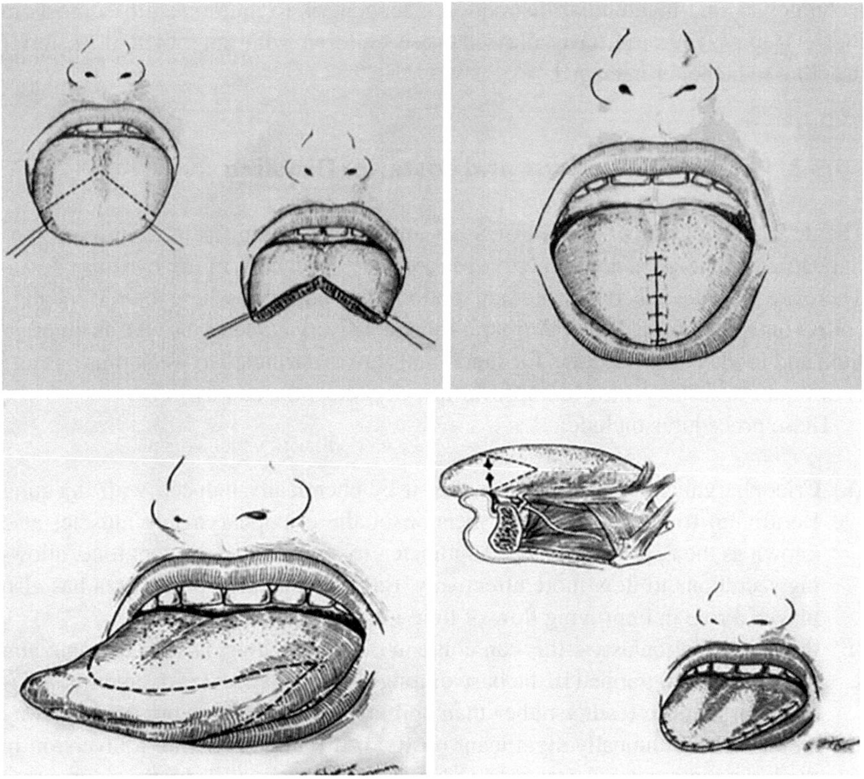

Fig. 10.1 Anterior tongue reduction surgery for paediatric macroglossia

the tongue base, hence increasing the retrolingual space during sleep, promoting lip closure and lessens drooling.

Transoral robotic surgery offers precise visualisation of the tongue base, and with the assistance of plasma-mediated ablation, base of tongue lingual tonsils can be precisely removed producing a safer alternative to managing children and adults with severe obstructive sleep apnoea. The technique is currently gathering momentum and is another research avenue that we should remain cognisant of, despite the concerns of safety and potential postoperative morbidity [32].

Plasma-mediated ablation is becoming an accepted method of lingual tonsil reduction and tongue base reduction given the very precise and localised nature of its effect. Given the 250 micron field of tissue clearance without thermal damage to the underlying lingual artery and its branches, it offers an acceptable form for this form of surgery [33]. It is particularly useful for children with lymphatic malformations residing in the floor of mouth and within tongue tissues.

The described literature on these patient groups has fostered ongoing treatment algorithms which have allowed creative and innovative strategies in managing drooling Posterior tongue base resection, the use of plasma-mediated ablative technologies and mandibular distraction osteogenesis to minimise glossoptosis in Pierre Robin syndrome have allowed these children with anterior and posterior drooling to be better managed.

10.3.3 Pharyngeal Residue and Posterior Drooling

The development of VFSS and FEES has allowed the clinicians to examine potential causes of the presence of pharyngeal residue especially in the pyriform fossa. There are well-described management options depending on where the residue may collect and predispose the child to aspiration of salivary contents, as well as ingested fluid and food. The procedures for functional causes attributed to weak muscles and coordination, surgery aims to improve flow or protect the airway [34].

These procedures include:

(a) Cricopharyngeal myotomy—whether it be chemically induced with injecting Botulinum toxin, or a precise incision of the cricopharyngeus muscle, also known as the upper oesophageal sphincter, to reduce the persistent tone, allowing secretions to flow more effectively. Balloon dilatation of the area has also played a role in improving flow of fluid into the oesophagus.
(b) Partial epiglottoplasty—this can come in differing forms, but the ultimate aim is to allow fluid trapped in the base of tongue or the valleculae to enter the pyriform fossa more readily rather than spilling over into the supraglottic airway which causes clinically significant posterior drooling. Creating a diversion in the laryngopharyngeal area may reduce pooling in the valleculae, or the act of lifting it up, and may cause secretions in the vallecula to spill more readily into the pyriform fossae.
(c) Pharyngeal augmentation or injection laryngoplasty has become a recent addition to the armamentarium of the swallowing surgeon, and the injection of materials such as fat, collagen or hyaluronic acid into the interarytenoid area has led to improvement in the child's ability to swallow and separates the laryngeal inlet from the pharyngeal inlet sufficiently to minimise posterior drooling [35].
(d) Laryngeal suspension or hyo-mandibular suspension—allows the supraglottic larynx to be lifted and makes the oesophagus easier to open.

In the case of severe chronic aspiration with no recourse, laryngotracheal separation allows disconnection of the larynx from the pharynx to prevent food entering the lungs. However, in the last 10 years, there are innovative methods used to increase the interarytenoid height of the posterior supraglottic airway, and this reduces the likelihood of aspiration as there is better timing and improved laryngeal sensation following surgical clearance of the intensely innervated supraglottic larynx [35]. There is also a growing realisation that the sensory pathways of the supraglottic airway, the key component to the laryngeal cough reflex, can be improved on with surgical division of the nerve fibres in the supra glottis. This can potentially re-sensitise the supra glottis, whose sensory fibres may have been blunted by gastro-oesophageal reflux, inflammation from other causes, the nasogastric tube syndrome or neurological immaturity in a child. There is increasing evidence that re-innervation surgery to the recurrent laryngeal nerve may have positive impact on the supraglottis via the Galen's anastomosis, which communicates the recurrent laryngeal nerve to the superior laryngeal nerve, and this is evidenced by the improved swallow reflexes of children who have had neurological insults from cardiothoracic surgery [36]. The improved swallowing has seen the children gain greater confidence, and this has improved the patient outcome scores of improved feeding and reduced drooling.

10.4 Conclusions

Chronic drooling in children is a symptom, and the underlying diagnosis requires a multidisciplinary approach. The contributing variates need to be fully understood before embarking on a combination of speech and swallowing therapy, pharmacotherapy and surgical options around the head and neck. In the past, allowing time and maturation to occur has been the mainstay of swallowing therapy in children. However, in the age of personalised medicine, the focus is on precision therapy using sophisticated technology, functional restoration and improving QOL for children and caregivers such that developmental delays are minimised.

References

1. Arvedson JC, Lefton-Greif MA. Pediatric swallowing and feeding: assessment and management. 3rd ed. San Diego: Plural Publishing; 2020.
2. Daniel M, Bailey S, Walker K, Hensley R, Badawi N, Cheng AT, Waters K. airway feeding and growth in infants with Robin sequence. Int J Pediatr Otorhinolaryngol. 2013;77(4):499–503.
3. Fairhurst CB, Cockerill H. Management of drooling in children. Arch Dis Child Educ Pract Ed. 2011;96(1):25–30.
4. Orriëns LB, de Groot SAF, van der Burg JJW, van den Hoogen FJA, van Hulst K, Erasmus CE. Interdisciplinary assessment and treatment of paediatric drooling: two decades of experience by the nijmegen saliva control team reflected in a stepwise algorithm. Eur J Pediatr. 2024;183(9):3979–85.
5. Sforza E, Onesimo R, Leoni C, Giorgio V, Proli F, Notaro F, Kuczynska EM, Cerchiari A, Selicorni A, Rigante D, Zampino G. Drooling outcome measures in paediatric disability: a systematic review. Eur J Pediatr. 2022;181(7):2575–92.
6. Speyer R, Cordier R, Kim JH, Cocks N, Michou E, Wilkes-Gillan S. Prevalence of drooling, swallowing, and feeding problems in cerebral palsy across the lifespan: a systematic review and meta-analyses. Dev Med Child Neurol. 2019;61(11):1249–58.
7. Delsing CP, Bekkers S, Erasmus CE, van Hulst K, van den Hoogen FJ. Posterior drooling in children with cerebral palsy and other neurodevelopmental disorders. Dev Med Child Neurol. 2021;63(9):1093–8.
8. Hughes A, Lambert EM. Drooling and aspiration of saliva. Otolaryngol Clin N Am. 2022;55(6):1181–94.

9. Koeken DCRM, van Hulst K, Lagarde MLJ, Pangalila RF, Erasmus CE, van den Engel-Hoek L. Validity, reliability and application of the paediatric posterior drooling scale. Child Care Health Dev. 2025;51(6):e70153.
10. van Hulst K, Jongerius PH, van den Hoogen FJA, Erasmus CE. Interdisciplinary assessment and treatment of paediatric drooling: two decades of experience reflected in a stepwise algorithm. Eur J Pediatr. 2024;183:2157–67.
11. Newman R, Vilardell N, Clavé P, Speyer R. Effect of bolus viscosity on swallowing safety and efficacy in neurological disorders: a systematic review. Dysphagia. 2016;31(2):232–49.
12. Messina F, Rocca S, Manca B, Scarponi L, Ninfa A, Schindler A, Pizzorni N. Pharyngeal residue scoring in fiberoptic endoscopic evaluation of swallowing: reliability comparison and applicability among different scales. Dysphagia. 2024;39(5):872–80.
13. Neubauer PD, Rademaker AW, Leder SB. The Yale pharyngeal residue severity rating scale: an anatomically defined and image-based tool. Dysphagia. 2015;30(5):521–8. https://doi.org/10.1007/s00455-015-9631-4. Epub 2015 Jun 7.
14. Gulati A, Kidane J, Chang JL. Patient reported outcome measures for salivary function: a systematic review. Laryngoscope. 2023;133(8):1796–805.
15. Reddihough D, Johnson H, Staples M, et al. Outcome measures for drooling in children with neurodevelopmental disabilities: a systematic review using COSMIN methodology. Dev Med Child Neurol. 2022;64(6):691–701.
16. Hadford SP, Genther DJ, Byrne PJ. Pediatric facial reanimation. Facial Plast Surg Clin North Am. 2024;32(1):169–80.
17. Lai M, Charters E, Low TH. Oral function in facial nerve palsy: a comparative analysis of flaccid and synkinetic palsy. J Plast Reconstr Aesthet Surg. 2025;106:435–42.
18. Movérare T, Lohmander A, Hultcrantz M, Sjögreen L. Peripheral facial palsy: speech, communication and oral motor function. Eur Ann Otorhinolaryngol Head Neck Dis. 2017;134(1):27–31. https://doi.org/10.1016/j.anorl.2015.12.002. Epub 2016 Nov 9.
19. Charters E, Coulson S. Oral competence following facial nerve paralysis: functional and quality of life measures. Int J Speech Lang Pathol. 2021;23(2):113–23.
20. Levi E, Alexander W, Cooper M. Management of paediatric sialorrhea. Curr Opin Otolaryngol Head Neck Surg. 2024;32(6):444–52. https://doi.org/10.1097/MOO.0000000000001015.
21. Hadlock TA, Greenfield LJ, Wernick-Robinson M, Cheney ML. Multimodality approach to management of the paralyzed face. Laryngoscope. 2006;116(8):1385–9.
22. Harrison DH. Surgical correction of unilateral and bilateral facial palsy. Postgrad Med J. 2005;81:562–7.
23. Ueda K, Harii K, Asato H, Yamada A. Neurovascular free muscle transfer combined with cross-face nerve grafting for the treatment of facial paralysis in children. Plast Reconstr Surg. 1998;101:1765–73.
24. McCrossan S, Martin S, Hill C. Tongue reduction for macroglossia. J Craniofac Surg. 2021;32(5):1856–9.
25. Kadouch DJ, Maas SM, Dubois L, van der Horst CM. Surgical treatment of macroglossia in patients with Beckwith-Wiedemann syndrome: a 20-year experience and review of the literature. Int J Oral Maxillofac Surg. 2012;41(3):300–8.
26. Brioude F, Kalish JM, Mussa A, et al. Expert consensus document: clinical and molecular diagnosis, screening and management of Beckwith-Wiedemann syndrome: an international consensus statement. Nat Rev Endocrinol. 2018;14(4):229–49.
27. Chau H, Soma M, Massey S, Hewitt R, Hartley B. Anterior tongue reduction surgery for paediatric macroglossia. J Laryngol Otol. 2011;125(12):1247–50.
28. Abraha B, MacIntyre O, Brennan H, Hong P, Bezuhly M. Outcomes of tongue reduction surgery in Beckwith-Wiedemann syndrome: a systematic review. J Craniofac Surg. 2025;36(2):542–6.
29. Shipster C, Morgan A, Dunaway D. Psychosocial, feeding, and drooling outcomes in children with Beckwith Wiedemann syndrome following tongue reduction surgery. Cleft Palate Craniofac J. 2012;49:25–34.

30. Serel Arslan S. Swallowing related problems of toddlers with down syndrome. J Dev Phys Disabil. 2022;12:1–11. https://doi.org/10.1007/s10882-022-09875-4. Epub ahead of print. PMID: 36118664; PMCID: PMC9465136.
31. Starmans JL, Bloem JJ. Tongreductie bij kinderen met het syndroom van down; een functionele operatie [tongue reduction in children with down's syndrome; a functional operation]. Ned Tijdschr Geneeskd. 1991;135(42):1963–6.
32. Lee JA, Byun YJ, Nguyen SA, Lentsch EJ, Gillespie MB. Transoral robotic surgery versus plasma ablation for Tongue Base reduction in obstructive sleep apnea: meta-analysis. Otolaryngol Head Neck Surg. 2020;162(6):839–52. https://doi.org/10.1177/0194599820913533. Epub 2020 Mar 24.
33. Roy S, Reyes S, Smith LP. Bipolar radio frequency plasma ablation (coblation) of lymphatic malformations of the tongue. Int J Ped Otorhinol. 2009;73:289–93.
34. Aldriweesh B, Alkhateeb A, Boudewyns A, Chan CY, Chun RH, El-Hakim HG, Fayoux P, Gerber ME, Kanotra S, Kaspy K, Kubba H, Lambert EM, Luscan R, Parikh SR, Rahbar R, Rickert SM, Russell J, Rutter M, Schroeder JW Jr, Schwarz Y, Sobol SE, Thevasagayam R, Thierry B, Thompson DM, Valika T, Watters K, Wei JL, Wyatt M, Zur KB, Daniel SJ. International pediatric otolaryngology group (IPOG) consensus on approach to aspiration. Int J Pediatr Otorhinolaryngol. 2024;176:111810.
35. Jefferson ND, Carmel E, Cheng AT. Low inter-arytenoid height: a subclassification of type 1 laryngeal cleft diagnosis and management. Int J Pediatr Otorhinolaryngol. 2015;79(1):31–5. https://doi.org/10.1016/j.ijporl.2014.10.040. Epub 2014 Nov 4.
36. Alahari S, Suresh R, Kline N, Liu P, Brown AF, Kou YF, Chorney SR, Johnson RF. Recurrent laryngeal nerve reinnervation and pediatric dysphagia outcomes. Laryngoscope Investig Otolaryngol. 2025;10(2):e70126.

GPSR Compliance

The European Union's (EU) General Product Safety Regulation (GPSR) is a set of rules that requires consumer products to be safe and our obligations to ensure this.

If you have any concerns about our products, you can contact us on ProductSafety@springernature.com

In case Publisher is established outside the EU, the EU authorized representative is:

Springer Nature Customer Service Center GmbH
Europaplatz 3
69115 Heidelberg, Germany

Batch number: 10370736

Printed by Printforce, the Netherlands